Michael B. Blank
Marlene M. Eisenberg
Editors

HIV:
Issues with Mental Health
and Illness

HIV: Issues with Mental Health and Illness has been co-published simultaneously as *Journal of Prevention & Intervention in the Community*, Volume 33, Numbers 1/2 2007.

"Much less well-understood or even discussed is the complex, multidirectional relationships between mental health status, HIV serostatus, HIV-related risk behaviors, and substance use. This volume–with chapters written by leaders in the field and expertly edited by Blank and Eisenberg–PROVIDES CRITICAL AND NEW INSIGHTS into these key relationships. . . . Blank, Eisenberg and the chapter authors, however, are not willing to merely describe public health challenges; they unveil interventions designed to address these challenges. From HIV prevention and treatment services for persons living with mental illness, to mental health services for persons in treatment for HIV disease, this volume PROVIDES KEY EXAMPLES AND IDEAS FOR STRENGTHENING PUBLIC HEALTH INTERVENTIONS AT THE INTERSECTION OF HIV AND MENTAL HEALTH. This book is rooted in the best principles of social epidemiology and public health action; IT DESERVES A PLACE THE LIBRARY OF ALL THOSE INTERESTED IN IMPROVING THE QUALITY OF LIFE OF PERSONS LIVING WITH HIV DISEASE, AND ALL THOSE INTERESTED IN PREVENTING HIV INFECTION."

David Holtgrave, PhD
Professor and Chair
Department of Health,
Behavior & Society
Bloomberg School of Public Health
Johns Hopkins University

"Since the earliest days of the epidemic we've known that HIV is connected directly with co-occuring epidemics such as substance abuse, depression, violence and other serious mental health problems. . . . Drs. Blank and Eisenberg have PROVIDED AN IMPORTANT SERVICE in their book *HIV: Issues with Mental Health and Illness* by focusing on how these interconnecting epidemics amplify each other and make treatment decisions more difficult."

Ron Stall, PhD, MPY
Professor and Assistant Dean
Graduate School of Public Health
University of Pittsburgh

HIV:
Issues with Mental Health and Illness

HIV: Issues with Mental Health and Illness has been co-published simultaneously as *Journal of Prevention & Intervention in the Community*, Volume 33, Numbers 1/2 2007.

Monographic Separates from the *Journal of Prevention & Intervention in the Community*®

For additional information on these and other Haworth Press titles, including descriptions, tables of contents, reviews, and prices, use the QuickSearch catalog at http://www.HaworthPress.com.

Journal of Prevention & Intervention in the Community is the successor title to *Prevention in Human Services,* which changed title after Vol. 12, No. 2 1995. *Journal of Prevention & Intervention in the Community,* under its new title, began with Volume 13, No. 1/2 1996.

HIV: Issues with Mental Health and Illness, edited by Michael B. Blank, PhD, and Marlene M. Eisenberg, PhD (Vol. 33, No. 1/2, 2007). ". . . . . *Deserves a place in the library of all those interested in improving the quality of life of persons living with HIV disease, and all those interested in preventing HIV infection.*" *(David Holtgrave, PhD, Professor and Chair, Department of Health, Behavior & Society, Bloomberg School of Public Health, Johns Hopkins University)*

Community Action Research: Benefits to Community Members and Service Providers, edited by Roger N. Reeb (Vol. 32, No. 1/2, 2006). *Detailed examination of empirical research that demonstrates the benefits of community action research for the 'at risk' community as well as the volunteers and paraprofessionals who implement community services.*

Creating Communities for Addiction Recovery: The Oxford House Model, edited by Leonard A. Jason, PhD, Joseph R. Ferrari, PhD, Margaret I. Davis, PhD, and Bradley D. Olson, PhD (Vol. 31, No. 1/2, 2006). *"This informative book is at once a systematic evaluation of an important intervention for addiction and a vivid illustration of the value of strengths-based community psychology research. Along the way, the authors show how the process of community research and the amount of knowledge it uncovers are enhanced by a respectful, dynamic relationship between academic scientists and community-based organizations." (Keith Humphreys, PhD, Associate Professor of Psychiatry, Stanford University)*

Psychological, Political, and Cultural Meanings of Home, edited by Mechthild Hart, PhD, and Miriam Ben-Yoseph, PhD (Vol. 30, No. 1/2, 2005). *Examines the meaning of home as a psychologically, spiritually, politically, or physically challenging experience.*

Technology Applications in Prevention, edited by Steven Godin, PhD, MPH, CHES (Vol. 29, No. 1/2, 2005). *Examines new prevention options made possible by today's cutting-edge technology.*

Six Community Psychologists Tell Their Stories: History, Contexts, and Narrative, edited by James G. Kelly, PhD, and Anna V. Song, MA (Vol. 28, No. 1/2, 2004). *"Should be required reading for any student aspiring to become a community psychologist as well as for practicing community psychologists interested in being provided unparalleled insights into the personal stories of many of the leading figures within our field. This book provides readers with an inside look at the reasons why a second generation of community psychologists entered this field, and also provides a rare glimpse of the excitement and passion that occured at some of the most important and dynamic community training settings over the past 40 years." (Leonard A. Jason, PhD, Professor of Psychology and Director, Center for Community Research, DePaul University)*

Understanding Ecological Programming: Merging Theory, Research, and Practice, edited by Susan Scherffius Jakes, PhD, and Craig C. Brookins, PhD (Vol. 27, No. 2, 2004). *Examines the background, concept, components, and benefits of using ecological programming in intervention/ prevention program designs.*

Leadership and Organization for Community Prevention and Intervention in Venezuela, edited by Maritza Montero, PhD (Vol. 27, No. 1, 2004). *Shows how (and why) participatory communities come into being, what they can accomplish, and how to help their leaders develop the skills they need to be most effective.*

Empowerment and Participatory Evaluation of Community Interventions: Multiple Benefits, edited by Yolanda Suarez-Balcazar, PhD, and Gary W. Harper, PhD, MPH (Vol. 26, No. 2, 2003). *"Useful . . . . Draws together diverse chapters that uncover the how and why of empowerment and participatory evaluation while offering exemplary case studies showing the challenges and successes of this community value-based evaluation model." (Anne E. Brodsky, PhD, Associate Professor of Psychology, University of Maryland Baltimore County)*

Traumatic Stress and Its Aftermath: Cultural, Community, and Professional Contexts, edited by Sandra S. Lee, PhD (Vol. 26, No. 1, 2003). *Explores risk and protective factors for traumatic stress, emphasizing the impact of cumulative/multiple trauma in a variety of populations, including therapists themselves.*

Culture, Peers, and Delinquency, edited by Clifford O'Donnell, PhD (Vol. 25, No. 2, 2003). *"Timely . . . . of value to both students and professionals. . . . Demonstrates how peers can serve as a pathway to delinquency from a multiethnic perspective. The discussion of ethnic, racial, and gender differences challenges the field to reconsider assessment, treatment, and preventative approaches." (Donald Meichenbaum, PhD, Distinguished Professor Emeritus, University of Waterloo, Ontario, Canada; Research Director, The Melissa Institute for Violence Prevention and the Treatment of Victims of Violence, Miami, Florida)*

Prevention and Intervention Practice in Post-Apartheid South Africa, edited by Vijé Franchi, PhD, and Norman Duncan, PhD, consulting editor (Vol. 25, No.1, 2003). *"Highlights the way in which preventive and curative interventions serve–or do not serve–the ideals of equality, empowerment, and participation. . . . Revolutionizes our way of thinking about and teaching socio-pedagogical action in the context of exclusion." (Dr. Altay A. Manço, Scientific Director, Institute of Research, Training, and Action on Migrations, Belgium)*

Community Interventions to Create Change in Children, edited by Lorna H. London, PhD (Vol. 24, No. 2, 2002). *"Illustrates creative approaches to prevention and intervention with at-risk youth . . . . Describes multiple methods to consider in the design, implementation, and evaluation of programs." (Susan D. McMahon, PhD, Assistant Professor, Department of Psychology, DePaul University)*

Preventing Youth Access to Tobacco, edited by Leonard A. Jason, PhD, and Steven B. Pokorny, PhD (Vol. 24, No. 1, 2002). *"Explores cutting-edge issues in youth access research methodology. . . . Provides a thorough review of the tobacco control literature and detailed analysis of the methodological issues presented by community interventions to increase the effectiveness of tobacco control. . . . Challenges widespread assumptions about the dynamics of youth access programs and the requirements for long-term success." (John A. Gardiner, PhD, LLB, Consultant to the 2000 Surgeon General's Report* Reducing Youth Access to Tobacco *and to the National Cancer Institute's evaluation of the ASSIST program)*

The Transition from Welfare to Work: Processes, Challenges, and Outcomes, edited by Sharon Telleen, PhD, and Judith V. Sayad (Vol. 23, No. 1/2, 2002). *A comprehensive examination of the welfare-to-work initiatives surrounding the major reform of United States welfare legislation in 1996.*

Prevention Issues for Women's Health in the New Millennium, edited by Wendee M. Wechsberg, PhD (Vol. 22, No. 2, 2001). *"Helpful to service providers as well as researchers . . . A useful ancillary textbook for courses addressing women's health issues. Covers a wide range of health issues affecting women." (Sherry Deren, PhD, Director, Center for Drug Use and HIV Research, National Drug Research Institute, New York City)*

Workplace Safety: Individual Differences in Behavior, edited by Alice F. Stuhlmacher, PhD, and Douglas F. Cellar, PhD (Vol. 22, No. 1, 2001). Workplace Safety: Individual Differences in Behavior *examines safety behavior and outlines practical interventions to help increase safety awareness. Individual differences are relevant to a variety of settings, including the workplace, public spaces, and motor vehicles. This book takes a look at ways of defining and measuring safety as well as a variety of individual differences like gender, job knowledge, conscientiousness, self-efficacy, risk avoidance, and stress tolerance that are important in creating safety interventions and improving the selection and training of employees.* Workplace Safety *takes an incisive look at these issues with a unique focus on the way individual differences in people impact safety behavior in the real world.*

HIV:
Issues with Mental Health and Illness

Michael B. Blank
Marlene M. Eisenberg
Editors

HIV: Issues with Mental Health and Illness has been co-published simultaneously as *Journal of Prevention & Intervention in the Community*, Volume 33, Numbers 1/2 2007.

The Haworth Press, Inc.

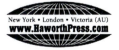

New York • London • Victoria (AU)
www.HaworthPress.com

MT

HIV: Issues with Mental Health and Illness has been co-published simultaneously as *Journal of Prevention & Intervention in the Community®*, Volume 33, Numbers 1/2 2007.

The development, preparation, and publication of this work has been undertaken with great care. However, the publisher, employees, editors, and agents of The Haworth Press and all imprints of The Haworth Press, Inc., including The Haworth Medical Press® and Pharmaceutical Products Press®, are not responsible for any errors contained herein or for consequences that may ensue from use of materials or information contained in this work. With regard to case studies, identities and circumstances of individuals discussed herein have been changed to protect confidentiality. Any resemblance to actual persons, living or dead, is entirely coincidental.

The Haworth Press is committed to the dissemination of ideas and information according to the highest standards of intellectual freedom and the free exchange of ideas. Statements made and opinions expressed in this publication do not necessarily reflect the views of the Publisher, Directors, management, or staff of The Haworth Press, Inc., or an endorsement by them.

Library of Congress Cataloging-in-Publication Data

HIV: issues with mental health and illness / Michael B. Blank, Marlene M. Eisenberg, editors.
  p. cm.
  "Co-published simultaneously as Journal of Prevention & Intervention in the Community, Volume 33, Numbers 1/2 2007."
  Includes bibliographical references and index.
  ISBN-13: 978-0-7890-3409-0 (hard cover : alk. paper)
  ISBN-10: 0-7890-3409-3 (hard cover : alk. paper)
  ISBN-13: 978-0-7890-3410-6 (soft cover : alk. paper)
  ISBN-10: 0-7890-3410-7 (soft cover : alk. paper)
  1. AIDS (Disease)–Patients–Mental health. 2. AIDS (Disease)–Psychological aspects. I. Blank, Michael B. II. Eisenberg, Marlene M. III. Journal of prevention & intervention in the community.
  [DNLM: 1. Acquired Immunodeficiency Syndrome–psychology. 2. Acquired Immunodeficiency Syndrome–prevention & control. 3. Mentally Ill Persons. 4. Community Mental Health Services.
W1 PR497 v.33 no.1-2 2007 / WC 503.7 H6766 2007]
RC606.6.H57 2007
362.196'9792–dc22

                           2006008536

2/1/06

The HAWORTH PRESS *Inc.*
Abstracting, Indexing & Outward Linking
PRINT *and* ELECTRONIC BOOKS & JOURNALS

This section provides you with a list of major indexing & abstracting services and other tools for bibliographic access. That is to say, each service began covering this periodical during the the year noted in the right column. Most Websites which are listed below have indicated that they will either post, disseminate, compile, archive, cite or alert their own Website users with research-based content from this work. (This list is as current as the copyright date of this publication.)

Abstracting, Website/Indexing Coverage . . . . Year When Coverage Began

- **Academic Search Premier (EBSCO)**
  <http://www.epnet.com/academic/acasearchprem.asp> 2006
- **CINAHL (Cumulative Index to Nursing & Allied Health Literature) (EBSCO)** *<http://www.cinahl.com>* 2006
- **CINAHL Plus (EBSCO)** 2006
- **MEDLINE (National Library of Medicine)** *<http://www.nlm.nih.gov>* 2005
- **Psychological Abstracts (PsycINFO)** *<http://www.apa.org>* 1998
- **PubMed** *<http://www.ncbi.nlm.nih.gov/pubmed/>* 2005
- **Social Services Abstracts (Cambridge Scientfic Abstracts)** *<http://csa.com>* 1998
- **Social Work Abstracts (NASW)** *<http://www.silverplatter.com/catalog/swab.htm>* 1996
- **Sociological Abstracts (Cambridge Scientific Abstracts)** *<http://www.csa.com>* 1998
- *Child Welfare Information Gateway (formerly National Adoption Information Clearinghouse Documents Database, and formerly National Adoption Information Clearinghouse on Child Abuse & Neglect Information Documents Database)* *<http://www.childwelfare.gov>* 2006
- *EBSCOhost Electronic Journals Service (EJS)* *<http://ejournals.ebsco.com>* 2001

(continued)

(continued)

*Exact start date to come.

Bibliographic Access

- *Cabell's Directory of Publishing Opportunities
  in Psychology <http://www.cabells.com>*

- *MediaFinder <http://www.mediafinder.com>*

- *Ulrich's Periodicals Directory: International Periodicals
  Information Since 1932 <http://www.Bowkerlink.com>*

*Special Bibliographic Notes related to special journal issues
(separates) and indexing/abstracting:*

- indexing/abstracting services in this list will also cover material in any "separate" that is co-published simultaneously with Haworth's special thematic journal issue or DocuSerial. Indexing/abstracting usually covers material at the article/chapter level.
- monographic co-editions are intended for either non-subscribers or libraries which intend to purchase a second copy for their circulating collections.
- monographic co-editions are reported to all jobbers/wholesalers/approval plans. The source journal is listed as the "series" to assist the prevention of duplicate purchasing in the same manner utilized for books-in-series.
- to facilitate user/access services all indexing/abstracting services are encouraged to utilize the co-indexing entry note indicated at the bottom of the first page of each article/chapter/contribution.
- this is intended to assist a library user of any reference tool (whether print, electronic, online, or CD-ROM) to locate the monographic version if the library has purchased this version but not a subscription to the source journal.
- individual articles/chapters in any Haworth publication are also available through the Haworth Document Delivery Service (HDDS).

As part of Haworth's continuing committment to better serve our library patrons, we are proud to be working with the following electronic services:

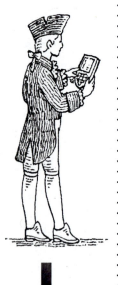

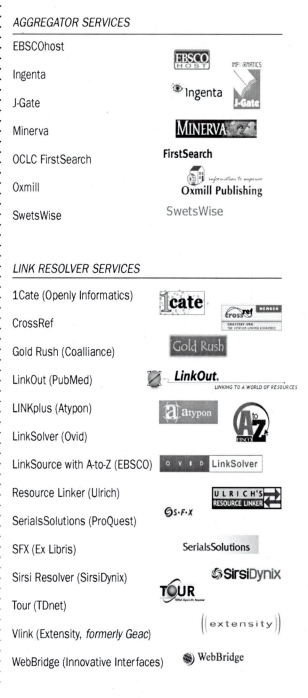

AGGREGATOR SERVICES

EBSCOhost

Ingenta

J-Gate

Minerva

OCLC FirstSearch

Oxmill

SwetsWise

LINK RESOLVER SERVICES

1Cate (Openly Informatics)

CrossRef

Gold Rush (Coalliance)

LinkOut (PubMed)

LINKplus (Atypon)

LinkSolver (Ovid)

LinkSource with A-to-Z (EBSCO)

Resource Linker (Ulrich)

SerialsSolutions (ProQuest)

SFX (Ex Libris)

Sirsi Resolver (SirsiDynix)

Tour (TDnet)

Vlink (Extensity, *formerly Geac*)

WebBridge (Innovative Interfaces)

HIV:
Issues with Mental Health and Illness

CONTENTS

ABOUT THE EDITORS

Michael B. Blank, PhD, is Assistant Professor of Psychology in Psychiatry at the University of Pennsylvania. Dr. Blank's research and writing focus on integration of health and mental health services delivery systems including treatment for co-morbid illness such as HIV/AIDS. Other areas of interest include informal care and its impact on consumers and families, rural mental health, ethics in prevention, and applications of technology and computer-assisted care in mental health service delivery. Dr. Blank's primary affiliation is with the Center for Mental Health Policy and Services Research in the Psychiatry Department. He also holds appointments as Senior Fellow at the Leonard Davis Institute for Health Economics, and the Schools of Nursing at the University of Pennsylvania and the University of Virginia.

Marlene M. Eisenberg, PhD, is Research Associate in Psychiatry at the University of Pennsylvania. Trained as a developmental psychologist, Dr. Eisenberg's current research focuses on substance abuse and HIV. Her research is concentrated in the area of public health and mental health services research with an additional focus on normative and clinical issues across the lifespan, intergenerational transmission of risk, mental health policy, and legal issues surrounding health related decision-making. Dr. Eisenberg's primary affiliation is with the Center for the Studies of Addiction at the University of Pennsylvania School of Medicine.

HIV and Mental Illness:
Opportunities for Prevention

Michael B. Blank

Marlene M. Eisenberg

University of Pennsylvania

The fields of public health and mental health have theoretically been collaborating since the beginnings of Community Psychology. However, the true integration of the two fields is only now being realized as viable public health interventions for HIV/AIDS take hold and the consequences of that disease as a chronic illness are observed within those diagnosed with serious mental illnesses. Mental health status not only mediates risk behaviors, but positive serostatus also has direct and indirect effects on mental health. The availability of more effective HIV treatments has reduced mortality, resulting in a growing number of people living with HIV, even as the incidence of new cases decreases in the United States. As such, a more complete understanding of the interactions between mental health status and HIV serostatus is of increasing importance.

Persons with mental illness have not traditionally been thought of as a group at risk for becoming infected with HIV in the same way as have other groups such as people who inject drugs, gay men, and people with multiple sex partners, but there is increasing recognition that mental illness makes people more vulnerable to contracting HIV and AIDS. This vulnerability is due in part to a disadvantaged social status and poverty which places them in contact with other high risk populations. Persons with mental illnesses have also been found to have higher rates of substance

[Haworth co-indexing entry note]: "HIV and Mental Illness: Opportunities for Prevention." Blank, Michael B., and Marlene M. Eisenberg. Co-published simultaneously in *Journal of Prevention & Intervention in the Community* (The Haworth Press, Inc.) Vol. 33, No.1/2, 2007, pp. 1-4; and: *HIV: Issues with Mental Health and Illness* (ed: Michael B. Blank, and Marlene M. Eisenberg) The Haworth Press, Inc., 2007, pp. 1-4. Single or multiple copies of this article are available for a fee from The Haworth Document Delivery Service [1-800-HAWORTH, 9:00 a.m. - 5:00 p.m. (EST). E-mail address: docdelivery@haworthpress.com].

Available online at http://jpic.haworthpress.com
doi:10.1300/J005v33n01_01

1

abuse, homelessness, homosexuality, and sex for sale, all of which are risk factors for infection with HIV/AIDS.

The prevalence of mental illness has also been found to be high among seropositive individuals. Co-morbid substance abuse is common among HIV positive individuals with severe mental illness, resulting in serious adverse effects. Evidence also shows that factors related to substance abuse in the general population such as being young, urban, male, single, and poorly educated also are predictive among persons with mental illnesses. Recent evidence shows that separate services for individuals with co-occurring substance abuse are less effective than treatment programs that integrate mental health and substance abuse. As well, any substance use at all compromises the effectiveness of mental health treatment.

With the inception of new pharmacotherapies and the advent of highly active retroviral therapy (HAART) drug regimens, a growing number of persons with HIV/AIDS have experienced greatly increased longevity and have joined the ranks of those living with a chronic illness. It is important to understand relationships between mental health and illness with HIV just as with other chronic illnesses, in order to help plan for reducing the number of persons affected by the epidemic, and to improve the mental health and quality of life of those who are HIV infected.

This volume is intended to provide an overview into the complex issues in HIV and mental health and illness. We have the privilege of presenting a collection of papers from a group of distinguished scholars and leading researchers. Many of them identify with community psychology and prevention, but others do not. We thought that breadth in presentation of issues in prevention and community intervention was more important than a narrow disciplinary focus. As such we have contributions from physicians, sociologists, nurses, social workers, as well as psychologists that represent a dovetailing of public health and mental health while presenting innovative research from a multi-disciplinary perspective.

The volume has three broad themes and the papers are roughly arranged accordingly. The first group focuses on clinical and diagnostic issues in mental health and HIV. The second group has to do with organization of service delivery systems and health and mental health services research in these populations. Finally, the last group of papers address themselves specifically to community-based preventive interventions including universal, selected, and indicated.

Among the papers addressing diagnostic and clinical issues, Jessy G. Dévieux, Robert Malow, Brenda G. Lerner, Janyce C. Dyer, Ligia Baptista, Barbara Lucenko, and Seth C. Kalichman raise issues related to what they describe as triple jeopardy for HIV infection; serious mental illness, alcohol and substance abuse, and lifetime exposure to trauma. They examine how these demographic factors can be useful in predicting HIV risk, and how targeted intervention should incorporate strategies for addressing multiple health risks. Next, Joachim G. Voss, Carmen J. Portillo, William L. Holzemer, and Marylin J. Dodd describe the interplay between depression, HIV, and chronic fatigue, as well difficulties in distinguishing between fatigue and depression. They emphasize the importance of distinguishing between depression and fatigue, and examine the sensitivity and specificity of a number of standardized instruments that can be used effectively in this population. They conclude that persons seeking treatment for either depression or fatigue should be evaluated for both conditions in order to develop tailored interventions. In the next paper, Margaret Shandor Miles, Diane Holditch-Davis, Cort Pedersen, Joseph J. Eron, Jr., and Todd Schwartz examine factors associated with increased emotional stress among a sample of African American women. They examine individual-level factors, cognitive and coping responses, and affective states in these women and identify factors related to increased concern about becoming HIV infected. Celia M. Lescano, Larry K. Brown, Paul M. Miller, and Kristie L. Puster follow with an examination of factors related to condom use among a sample of adolescents with psychiatric disorders. They find that self-efficacy for condom use while distressed was predictive of reports of consistent condom use in this group, and draw some conclusions about the implications for how clinical practice can be enhanced for adolescents.

The next group of papers specifically addresses how service delivery can and should be modified to address needs of those with mental illness and at risk for HIV and other STIs. They address issues in best practice models in mental health service delivery systems, and how these systems can be enhanced to address HIV prevention. In the first paper, Eric R. Wright, Dustin E. Wright, and Anthony H. Lawson examine five public mental health care programs in order to examine what are current practices about providing HIV prevention services to adults with serious mental illnesses. They conclude that client gender as well as type of service setting influenced the types and frequency of preventive services offered. Next, Peter A. Vanable, Michael P. Carey, Kate B. Carey, and Stephen A. Maisto provide a comprehensive examination of those receiving community-based services for a mental illness who did and did not have a history of a sexually transmitted infection (STI) in order to begin to develop an understanding of how HIV knowledge, attitudes, and behaviors differ among these groups. Their findings provide compelling evidence for the need to integrate interventions designed to address STI risk reduction strategies into ongoing community mental health treatment. In the next paper, James Satriano, Karen McKinnon, and Spencer Adoff present findings from their survey of the types of HIV services offered in 1997 to persons with mental illnesses in outpatient care settings in New York. They emphasize the need to integrate HIV prevention services into mental health care, since they found that virtually the only health care received was through mental health providers. This finding only highlights the need for better integration of primary care and specialty mental health services for those with mental illnesses. In the next paper, Seth Himelhoch, Neil R. Powe, William Breakey, and Kelly A. Gebo use data from a national survey of HIV clinicians in order to examine how co-morbid schizophrenia influences the decision to provide HAART therapy. Their findings indicate that clinicians were as likely to prescribe antiretrovirals for those with schizophrenia, and they were reluctant to prescribe medications with known neuropsychiatric side effects. They examine both these issues from an individual-, clinical- and a population-based perspective.

The third group of papers reflects the fledgling area of community-based preventive interventions for HIV/AIDS among persons with mental illnesses. In the first paper, Kathleen J. Sikkema, Christina S. Meade, Jhan D. Doughty-Berry, Susan O. Zimmerman, Bret Kloos, and David L. Snow describe implementing such a program within the context of a supported housing program. This innovation is particularly well conceived given the frequency of homelessness among persons with mental illness and the concomitant risks that accompany homelessness. The final paper in this collection addresses and ecological assessment of a mental health clinic to assess readiness for implementation of an HIV prevention program by Phyllis L. Solomon, Julie A. Tennille, David Lipsitt, Ellen Plumb, David Metzger, and Michael B. Blank. This paper describes a rapid assessment procedure that is preceding implementation of a comprehensive HIV prevention program for persons with mental illness delivered by their case managers. Findings indicated that consumers, front line staff, and administrators all had different viewpoints on the availability of HIV preventive services, but that they agreed that more services were needed within community mental health systems of care.

It has been a pleasure for us to interact with the authors that contributed to this volume, and to help shape its development. We see this as auguring a new era in mental health and prevention science. This era can be one that integrates public health and public mental health utilizing what we know about prevention science to maximize the impact of our efforts and improve the quality of life in our communities.

Triple Jeopardy for HIV: Substance Using Severely Mentally Ill Adults

Jessy G. Dévieux
Robert Malow
Brenda G. Lerner
Janyce G. Dyer

Florida International University

Ligia Baptista

Edith Nourse Rogers Memorial Veterans Administration Hospital

Barbara Lucenko

Washington State Center for Court Research

Seth C. Kalichman

University of Connecticut

SUMMARY. Severely Mentally Ill (SMI) adults have disproportionately high HIV seroprevalence rates. Abuse of alcohol and other sub-

---

Address correspondence to: Jessy G. Dévieux, Florida International University, College of Health and Urban Affairs, Stempel School of Public Health, Biscayne Bay Campus ACI-260, 3000 NE 151st Street, North Miami, FL 33181.

This research was supported in part by the National Institute on Alcohol Abuse and Alcoholism (NIAAA) Grant: RO1AA12115.

[Haworth co-indexing entry note]: "Triple Jeopardy for HIV: Substance Using Severely Mentally Ill Adults." Dévieux, Jessy G. et al. Co-published simultaneously in *Journal of Prevention & Intervention in the Community* (The Haworth Press, Inc.) Vol. 33, No.1/2, 2007, pp. 5-18; and: *HIV: Issues with Mental Health and Illness* (ed: Michael B. Blank, and Marlene M. Eisenberg) The Haworth Press, Inc., 2007, pp. 5-18. Single or multiple copies of this article are available for a fee from The Haworth Document Delivery Service [1-800-HAWORTH, 9:00 a.m. - 5:00 p.m. (EST). E-mail address: docdelivery@haworthpress.com].

stances (AOD) and lifetime exposure to trauma by others are particularly potent risk factors, which, in combination with psychiatric disabilities, create triple jeopardy for HIV infection. This study examined the predictive utility of demographic characteristics; history of physical, emotional, or sexual abuse; extent of drug and alcohol abuse; knowledge about HIV/AIDS; sexual self-efficacy; and condom attitudes toward explaining the variance in a composite of HIV high-risk behavior among 188 SMI women and 158 SMI men. History of sexual abuse, engaging in sexual activities while high on substances, and lower cannabis use were the most significant predictors of HIV sexual risk behaviors. Given the triple jeopardy for HIV risk in this population, a triple barreled approach that simultaneously addresses multiple health risks within an integrated treatment setting is warranted. doi:10.1300/J005v33n01_02 *[Article copies available for a fee from The Haworth Document Delivery Service: 1-800-HAWORTH. E-mail address: <docdelivery@haworthpress.com> Website: <http://www.HaworthPress.com> © 2007 by The Haworth Press, Inc. All rights reserved.]*

KEYWORDS. Severely mentally ill, HIV risk, trauma, sexual abuse and HIV risk

Severely mentally ill (SMI) adults or individuals suffering from persistent and serious psychiatric symptoms and conditions show disproportionately high and escalating HIV seroprevalence rates (Carey, Weinhardt, & Carey, 1995; Rosenberg et al., 2001). These rates have been linked to a nexus of interacting clinical, behavioral, and contextual factors (Cournos & McKinnon, 1997; Kelly, 1997; Otto-Salaj, Kelly, Stevenson, Hoffman, & Kalichman, 2001).

Abuse of alcohol and other substances (AOD) have clearly been identified as potent risk factors for the development of HIV infection (Dausey & Desai, 2003). Nearly half of SMI individuals will develop some type of substance use disorder within their lifetime (RachBeisel, Scott, & Dixon, 1999; Regier et al., 1990). Those SMI adults who are dually diagnosed with a substance use disorder are at significantly greater risk for HIV infection than individuals with a single psychiatric diagnosis (Carey et al., 2004; McKinnon & Cournos, 1998). In combination with psychiatric disability, AOD can exacerbate psychotic symptoms and impede judgment and impulse control, leading to higher risk for HIV by increasing sexual desire, lowering sexual inhibition, and/or disturbing the consistent practice of safer sex.

Lifetime traumatic abuse by others has a substantial impact on risk behaviors for both genders. Sexual and/or physical assault histories have been associated with high-risk sexual practices in AOD abusing women (Dansky, Saladin, Brady, Kilpatrick, & Resnick, 1995; Hien & Scheier, 1996), in SMI women (Rosenberg, Drake, & Mueser, 1996), and in a community sample of both males and females (Bensley, Eenwyk, & Simmons, 1999). AOD abusing women who are also severely mentally ill have high rates of traumatic abuse histories (Malow et al., in press). Traumatic abuse severity is also positively correlated with HIV risk (Malow et al., in press). Thus, by virtue of the heightened risk for HIV that is associated with membership in three separate but underserved groups (SMI, AOD, victims of traumatic abuse by others), SMI adults appear to be at triple jeopardy for HIV infection. Within the cognitive-behavioral realm, information processing deficits that are an inherent component of the symptoms associated with SMI substance abusers, coupled with lack of knowledge and misconceptions about HIV transmission, may be mediating factors that contribute to HIV risk among SMI adults (Aruffo, Coverdale, Chacko, & Dworkin, 1990; Kalichman, Kelly, Johnson, & Bulto, 1994; Kelly & Murphy, 1992). However, other studies with SMI adults have shown that adequate amounts of HIV related knowledge is partially independent of HIV risk behavior but that knowledge by itself is not sufficient to explain behavior (McKinnon, Cournos, Sugden, Guido, & Herman, 1996).

SMI substance abusers present distinctive risks by virtue of their comorbidities and the attendant contextual challenges to cognitive and behavioral change. However, there is a paucity of information on the linkages between these risks. In order to determine what constitutes high-risk behavior in this population, we sought to identify a composite of experiences related to the practice of unsafe sex and sexual relations with high-risk partners. Thus, we examined the predictive utility of demographic characteristics; history of physical, emotional, or sexual abuse; extent of drug and alcohol abuse; knowledge of HIV/AIDS; sexual self-efficacy; and condom attitudes toward explaining the variance in HIV high-risk behavior among inner-city SMI adults in outpatient treatment.

METHOD

Participants

Of the 346 participants, 188 (54.3%) were women and 158 (45.7%) were men attending day and residential mental health treatment at 16 psychiatric or combined addiction mental health programs in the metropolitan Miami-Dade area. Participants were identified from 444 individuals who volunteered to be screened for the study; there were 126 exclusions. The study exclusion criteria were: (a) residency outside of Miami-Dade, Florida (n = 31); (b) transportation difficulties that would preclude participation; (c) non-English speaking primary language (n = 5); (d) denial of drug or alcohol use in the past 6 months (n = 36); (e) did not meet criteria for severe mental illness (n = 3); and, (f) evidence of severe cognitive dysfunction as indicated by inability to concentrate or focus during screening session or intake assessment (n = 14). Seven participants left their respective treatment centers and 30 of those eligible refused to participate in the study.

Assessment Procedures

All assessment procedures were conducted by seasoned interviewers, trained to create a process sensitive to gender and cultural issues as well as to adopt a nonjudgmental attitude to establish rapport and build trust. To prevent interviewer drift and other contaminating factors, assessors received ongoing supervision from a clinical psychologist throughout the study. Following informed consent, assessment measures were verbally administered to facilitate full completion and to compensate for any literacy difficulties. In the event that a respondent showed any confusion, an assessor would repeat or elaborate on questions.

A manual and a procedural checklist were used to ensure standard administration of the assessment measures. Interviews were performed in a private room to guarantee confidentiality and enhance compliance. Interviewers used key events and calendar time lines to facilitate accurate reporting of the participants' behavior over the recall period.

Measures

Psychiatric Diagnoses. Researchers abstracted current Axis I and Axis II diagnoses based on the fourth edition of the Diagnostic and Statistical Manual of Mental Disorders (DSM-IV) (APA, 1994) from participants' clinical records at study sites. Most current chart diagnoses were taken as the best approximation of diagnosis at the time of data collection.

Abuse History Questionnaire. This instrument evaluated lifetime prevalence of abuse. All respondents were asked, "In your lifetime, have you ever been (a) sexually abused, (b) emotionally abused, and/or (c) physically abused?" Direct questions were used to assess abuse history to allow participants to self-define abuse situations rather than narrowly defining specific abuse events.

The Addiction Severity Index (ASI). This comprehensive, structured clinical research interview was selected to gather sociodemographic information (i.e., age, self-identified ethnic background, years of education, marital status, and employment status), psychiatric history and current symptoms, and alcohol and drug abuse history (McLellan, Metzger, & Peters, 1992). The ASI has shown high concurrent and inter-rater reliability (.74 to .93) and validity among a similar sample of SMI adults. Furthermore, drug treatment outcome research has repeatedly used the ASI and has found it to be reliable, valid, and effective in evaluating adults with serious mental illness (Zanis, McLellan, Cnaan, & Randall, 1994).

The AIDS Risk Reduction Model Questionnaire Revised (ARRM-QR). The ARRM-QR was created to reliably and validly measure the cognitive behavioral constructs that the ARRM model hypothesizes to be predictive of HIV-risk behaviors (Catania, Kegeles, & Coates, 1990). Subscales used in the present study to predict level of HIV-risk included: knowledge about HIV and AIDS, sexual self-efficacy, anxiety about contracting HIV, and condom attitudes. Scoring for the knowledge about HIV and AIDS subscale was based on the summed total of correct answers with a maximum total score of 18. The scales for condom attitudes, sexual self-efficacy, and anxiety subscale had a 4-point Likert format with response options ranging from 1 (*strongly disagree*) to 4 (*strongly agree*). For each scale, higher scores reflect a more positive response.

Risk Behavior Assessment (RBA) (National Institute on Drug Abuse, 1991). Participants reported the number of male and female sexual partners, intercourse frequency with men and women, and number of times condoms were used during vaginal and anal sex in the past three months. A three-month time frame has been shown to generate reliable recall of sexual behaviors (Kauth, St. Lawrence, & Kelly, 1991). In addition, we asked participants to report (a) number of sex partners, (b) number of occasions of sexual activity, and (c) consistency of condom use during intercourse. Participants described their sexual behavior with primary, casual, and/or "trading" sex partners. A primary sex partner was defined as a person with whom the respondent had a current or long-term relationship. Casual partners were defined as people with whom the respondent had sex, but with limited emotional involvement. A "trading" relationship was characterized by encounters in which sex was exchanged for money or drugs, whether received or given. The RBA has shown adequate test-retest reliability for sexual risk behaviors (Needle et al., 1995) and is similar to instruments used in past research to assess sexual behavior in adults diagnosed with SMI (Kalichman et al., 1994).

Levels of HIV Risk Behavior Composite. This scale was derived from six dichotomous items from the RBA that assessed the presence or absence of HIV risk factors for the preceding three months. Risk factors included: (a) having injection drug using partner, (b) sex with homosexual man, (c) engaging in sexual trade (e.g., sex for shelter, money, drugs), (d) unprotected vaginal or anal sex, (e) more than one partner, and (f) occurrence of STDs. These factors were summed to estimate HIV risk based on a continuous index, in which multiple factors indicate higher risk.

Data Analysis

Multiple regression analysis was utilized to test for the influence of the predictors on the levels of HIV risk behavior composite. A hierarchical analysis with sets of variables was used with predictors entered sequentially in four blocks (Cohen & Cohen, 1983). Sets of variables were added cumulatively to the equation in an order that approximated their temporal relationship to the HIV high-risk related behaviors. The variables of gender, age, and ethnicity were entered in the first block to examine preexisting demographic differences that could account for the variance in the risk composite. Lifetime history of emotional, physical, and sexual abuse was entered in the second block. Drug use variables were entered into the third block including number of times alcohol, marijuana, heroin, and cocaine were used in the last 30 days, as well as frequency of sex while high. Knowledge of HIV/AIDS, anxiety regarding contraction of HIV/AIDS, condom attitudes, and sexual self-efficacy were entered in the fourth block. This order controls for demographics, introduces traumatic abuse and substance abuse as independent blocks of indicators, and finally enters variables that are the target of cognitive-behavioral risk reduction interventions.

RESULTS

Description of the Sample

Based on the distributions of participant self-report and clinic charts, the modal sample participant was an indigent, ethnic minority individual who was diagnosed with schizophrenia, abused alcohol, non-injection "crack" cocaine and/or marijuana, and lived in the urban inner city. The participants ranged in age from 19 to 81 years ($M = 58.01$, $SD = 12.18$), and years of formal education ranged from 0 to 18 years, with 41.3% having completed high school. Their marital status distribution was as follows: single, 52%; married, 7%; separated/divorced, 36%; and widowed, 5%. Approximately 55% of participants were unemployed. Participants were 50.9% African American; 26.3% Non-Hispanic White; 20.8% Hispanic or Cuban, South American, Mexican or Puerto Rican origin; and 2% of other ethnic origin (i.e., Asian, Native American). The most common psychiatric diagnosis for the sample was schizophrenia (23%), followed by major depressive disorder (19%). Clinic chart diagnostic data were missing on 28 participants. Of the remaining participants, 92% had a major psychiatric disorder, while 46% of participants met criteria for both substance abuse/dependence and psychiatric disorder. Emotional, physical, or sexual abuse was a common phenomenon in this sample with 76% ($n = 262$) of participants reporting abuse of some form. For the entire sample, 68% ($n = 236$) had been emotionally abused, 53% ($n = 186$) had been physically abused, and 41% ($n = 141$) had been sexually abused. Multiple abuse experiences were frequent, with 26% ($n = 91$) of participants reporting two forms of abuse and 30% ($n = 105$) of participants reporting three forms of abuse.

Average use of substances in the previous 30 days was reported as follows: alcohol, 6.77 times ($SD = 11.18$); cannabis, 2.40 times ($SD = 7.32$); cocaine, 2.18 times ($SD = 6.85$); and heroin, 0.62 times ($SD = 4.05$). Mean scores on the cognitive behavioral constructs were as follows: knowledge of HIV/AIDS ($M = 13.27$, $SD = 3.07$), attitudes towards using condoms ($M = 3.23$, $SD = .42$), sexual self-efficacy ($M = 3.02$, $SD = .53$), and anxiety about contacting AIDS ($M = 3.01$, $SD = .74$). There were no significant differences between treatment sites on the levels of risk composite ($F(3,219) = .302$, $p = .82$).

HIV Risk Behaviors

Table 1 shows frequency and relative percentages of HIV sexual risk behavior for men and women in this sample. The most frequent risk behavior for both men ($n = 68$) and women ($n = 105$) was having unprotected vaginal or anal sex during the last 30 days. The average number of risk factors per participant was 1.31 ($SD = 1.24$) and ranged from none (33.2%) to six (.3%). Results were analyzed using bivariate correlations and multiple regression. The highest significant correlations among the variables include alcohol use and cocaine use ($r = .40$), cannabis use and alcohol use ($r = .35$), cannabis use and cocaine use ($r = .44$), sexual self-efficacy and condom attitudes ($r = .49$), history of physical abuse and history of emo-

TABLE 1. HIV Risk Behaviors Composite by Gender

Variable	Males $n = 158$	Females $n = 188$
IV Drug Use	2 (1.26%)	3 (1.60%)
Sex with an MSM	11 (6.96%)	13 (6.91%)
Sex for Trade	37 (23.42%)	52 (27.66%)
Unprotected Vaginal or Anal Intercourse	68 (43.04%)	105 (55.85%)
Sex with Multiple Partners	51 (32.28%)	71 (37.77%)
History of STDs in past 30 days	14 (8.86%)	27 (14.36%)

tional abuse ($r = .50$), and history of sexual abuse and history of emotional abuse ($r = .40$). We found no evidence of multicollinearity among the predictors or violations of other assumptions of regression.

Predicting HIV Risk Behaviors

Table 2 displays the unstandardized regression coefficients (B), the standardized regression coefficients (β), and R, R^2 and adjusted R^2 after entry of all four blocks of predictors. The variables in the first block did not contribute significantly to predicting level of HIV risk. The inclusion of history of abuse variables in the second block contributed significantly to predicting risk, with blocks 1 and 2 combined accounting for approximately 5% of the variance. The standardized regression coefficients show that lifetime history of sexual abuse contributed the most among variables in the second block. The inclusion of drug use variables in block 3 also considerably contributed to predicting HIV risk, accounting for approximately 23% of the variance. Examining the standardized regression coefficients for the third block illustrates that drug use during sexual intercourse and frequency of cannabis use over the last 30 days contributed the most among variables in this block. To identify the role that cognitive-behavioral constructs have on predicting risk level, we entered knowledge of HIV/AIDS, condom attitudes, sexual self-efficacy, and

TABLE 2. Hierarchical Regression Predicting Level of Risk Composite

Variables	B	β	t	ΔR^2
Block 1				
Sex	.08	.03	.64	
Non-Hispanic White Ethnicity	−.23	−.08	−1.43	
Hispanic	−.11	−.04	−.67	
Other Ethnicity	.08	.01	.20	
Age	−.006	−.07	−1.35	.018
Block 2				
History of Emotional Abuse	−.05	−.02	−.35	
History of Physical Abuse	.14	.05	.96	
History of Sexual Abuse	.32	.13	2.28*	.028
Block 3				
Sex When High on Drugs	1.24	.46	8.99***	
Alcohol Use Last 30 Days	−.009	.09	1.68	
Heroin Use Last 30 Days	−.01	−.04	−.88	
Cocaine Use Last 30 Days	.009	.06	.95	
Cannabis Use Last 30 Days	−.02	−.16	−2.82**	.227
Block 4				
Knowledge	−.02	.06	1.03	
Condom Attitudes	−.21	−.07	−1.23	
Sexual Self-Efficacy	−.04	−.02	−.33	
Anxiety	.07	.04	.88	.007
Constant	1.47		2.47*	
				R^2 = .28
				Adj. R^2 = .24 R = .53

*$p \leq .05$ **$p \leq .01$ ***$p \leq .001$

anxiety about contracting HIV/AIDS variables into the fourth block. In the final model, history of sexual abuse ($\beta = .13, t = 2.28, p = .023$), being high during sex ($\beta = .47, t = 8.99, p < .001$), and lower cannabis use in the last month ($\beta = -.13, t = -2.82, p = .005$) significantly predicted a greater level of HIV risk behaviors ($R^2 = .28, F(17, 328) = 7.52, p < .001$).

DISCUSSION

These findings demonstrate that in a sample of inner city, ethnically diverse SMI adults from a variety of mental health and substance abuse treatment sites, history of sexual abuse, greater frequency of substance use while engaging in sex and lower cannabis use are most predictive of HIV risk. We also found that SMI adults demonstrated a variety of highly risky sexual behaviors including unprotected vaginal or anal sex, sex for money or drugs, sex with multiple partners, and history of STDs. Other correlates of HIV risk behavior such as age, gender, ethnicity, knowledge about HIV/AIDS, anxiety regarding contraction of HIV/AIDS, attitudes toward condom use, and sexual self-efficacy were not predictive.

The findings establishing a link between sexual abuse and high-risk behaviors are consistent with those from other studies that link past sexual trauma with subsequent sexual maladjustment and increased engagement in sexual risk behaviors (Miller, 1999). History of sexual abuse has also been repeatedly linked to substance use/abuse (Burnam et al., 1988; Finkelhor, Hotaling, Lewis, & Smith, 1990) as well as to HIV risk behavior (Malow et al., in press), further supporting the notion that abuse trauma may be mediated by substance use in subsequent HIV risk behavior. In the aftermath of sexual trauma, it may be that drugs are used as a coping mechanism, which subsequently increases the likelihood of engaging in sexual risk behavior through disinhibition or dissociation (Miller, 1999).

A high prevalence of sexual abuse has been noted in the SMI literature. Mueser, Goodman, and Trumbetta (1998) reported that among a sample of SMI adults, 35% of men and 52% of women had experienced child sexual abuse compared to 16% and 27% respectively in the general population. Forty percent of the study participants in the current study reported a lifetime history of sexual abuse. Of this subgroup, three-fourths were women and one-fourth were men. Sexual trauma has been related to a variety of negative outcomes in SMI adults such as more severe symptoms, greater use of substances, and higher rates of posttraumatic stress disorder (PTSD), a common comorbid disorder in SMI adults (Mueser et al., 1998; Rosenberg et al., 2001). It has been theorized that PTSD may mediate the negative effects of sexual trauma on the course of SMI and subsequent HIV risk both directly, through the effects of specific symptoms of PTSD (i.e., avoidance, overarousal, and re-experiencing the trauma) and indirectly, through the effects of correlates of PTSD (i.e., retraumatization, substance abuse, and difficulties with interpersonal relationships) (Mueser, Rosenberg, Goodman, & Trumbetta, 2002).

Unprotected and risky sexual practices as a long-term consequence of sexual abuse are also found in populations who do not have the cognitive impairments manifested in SMI adults (Bensely et al., 1999; Cunningham, Stiffman, Doreˊ, & Earles, 1994). Thus, it may be that the potency of the trauma may overshadow any other factors that might moderate the relationship between sexual abuse and HIV risk behaviors.

This finding also suggests that those who have experienced sexual abuse may have great difficulties in initiating and carrying out safer sexual behaviors. Using drugs as part of their sexual experience may be a form of self-treatment that offers immediate relief from the impact of abuse. Interestingly, in our sample there was a negative relationship between cannabis use and HIV sexual risk behaviors. It could be conjectured that cannabis provides less of a feeling of disinhibition than alcohol or cocaine.

Given the triple jeopardy for HIV risk in this sample, a triple barreled approach that simultaneously addresses multiple risks within an integrated treatment setting is a necessity for HIV prevention efforts. The participants in this study represented a severely impaired group in terms of psychiatric diagnoses, degree of substance use and abuse, and rates of sexual abuse. Any targeted HIV prevention interventions should include both sexual and substance abuse risk reduction approaches (Carey et al., 2004) against the backdrop of psychiatric comorbidities. Because of the lack of association between the cognitive-behavioral constructs and HIV risk behaviors, other factors need to be considered such as specific symptom clusters that are more closely tied to cognitions; differential responses based on diagnosis; or, the impact on information processing by such factors as disinhibition or dissociation. Interventions targeted for this population may need to be tailored specifically to the patient's level of functioning as well as diagnostic category (Carey, Carey, Maisto, Gordon et al., 2004).

In light of the implications for designing interventions to reduce the spread of HIV and other STDs among SMI adults, certain limitations should be noted in interpretation of the findings. One concern in developing the risk composite was the possibility of correlation between variables, both within the composite and the overlap between predictors. For example, it is very likely that our model did not account for or masked naturally occurring combined practices such as use of cocaine with sex trade because of the need to barter drugs for money/housing (i.e., "survival sex").

The reliance on clinical records for psychiatric diagnoses and self-report for substance use and sexual behavior raise reliability concerns, and pertinent findings should thus be interpreted with caution. The direct or indirect contribution of specific psychiatric symptoms cannot be determined from these analyses. Future studies addressing risk behavior among SMI adults should focus on specific symptomatology and comorbidity with PTSD in predicting risk and as mediating factors in HIV prevention interventions. This would increase the ecological validity and enhance implications for assessment and risk prevention.

REFERENCES

American Psychiatric Association: *Diagnostic and statistical manual of mental disorders* (4th ed.). Washington, DC: Author, 1994.

Aruffo, J. F., Coverdale, J. H., Chacko, R. C., & Dworkin, R. J. (1990). Knowledge about AIDS among women psychiatric outpatients. *Hospital and Community Psychiatry, 41*, 326-328.

Bensley, L. S., Eenwyk, J. V., & Simmons, K. (1999). Self-reported childhood sexual and physical abuse and adult HIV-risk behaviors and heavy drinking. *American Journal of Preventive Medicine 18*, 151-158.

Burnham, M.A., Stein, M.A., Golding, J.M., Siegel, J.M., Sorenson, S.B., Forsythe, A.B. et al. (1988). Sexual assault and mental disorders in a community population. *Journal of Consulting and Clinical Psychology, 56*, 843-850.

Carey, M.P., Carey, K.B., Maisto, S.A., Gordon, C.M., Schroder, K.E.E., & Vanable, P.A. (2004). Reducing HIV-risk behavior among adults receiving outpatient psychiatric treatment: Results from a randomized controlled trial. *Journal of Consulting and Clinical Psychology, 72*(2), 252-268.

Carey, M.P., Carey, K.B., Maisto, S.A., Schroder, K.E.E., Vanable, P.A., & Gordon, C.M. (2004). HIV risk behavior among psychiatric outpatients: Association with psychiatric disorder, substance use disorder, and gender. *The Journal of Nervous and Mental Disease, 192*(4), 289-296.

Carey, M. P., Weinhardt, L. S., & Carey, K. B. (1995). Prevalence of infection with HIV among the seriously mentally ill: Review of research and implications for practice. *Professional Psychology: Research and Practice, 26*, 262-268.

Catania, J. A., Kegeles, S. M., & Coates, T. J. (1990). Towards an understanding of risk behavior: An AIDS risk reduction model (ARRM). *Health Education Quarterly, 17*, 53-72.

Cohen, J., & Cohen, P. (1983). *Applied multiple regression/correlation analysis for the behavioral sciences.* Hilldale, NJ: Laurence Erlbaum Associates.

Cournos, F., & McKinnon, K. (1997) Substance use and HIV risk among people with severe mental illness. *NIDA Research Monograph, 172*, 110-129.

Cunningham, R., Stiffman, A.R., Dore´, P., & Earles, F. (1994). The association of physical and sexual abuse with HIV risk behaviors in adolescence and young adulthood: Implications for public health. *Child Abuse & Neglect, 18*(3), 233-245.

Dansky, B.S., Saladin, M.E., Brady, K.T., Kilpatrick, D.G., & Resnick, H.S. (1995). Prevalence of victimization and posttraumatic stress disorders: Comparison of telephone and in-person assessment samples. *International Journal of Addictions, 30*(9), 1079-99.

Dausey, D.J., & Desai, R.A. (2003). Psychiatric comorbidity and the prevalence of HIV infection in a sample of patients in treatment for substance abuse. *The Journal of Nervous and Mental Disease, 191*(1), 10-17.

Finkelhor, D., Hotaling, G., Lewis, L.A. & Smith, C. (1990). Sexual abuse in a national survey of adult men and women: Prevalence, characteristics and risk factors. *Child Abuse & Neglect, 14*,19-28.

Hien, D., & Scheier, J. (1996). Trauma and short-term outcome for women in detoxification. *Journal of Substance Abuse Treatment, 13*(3), 227-231.

Kalichman, S. C., Kelly, J. A., Johnson, J. R., & Bulto, M. (1994). Factors associated with risk for HIV infection among chronic mentally ill adults. *American Journal of Psychiatry, 151,* 221-227.

Kauth, M., St. Lawrence, J. S., & Kelly, J. A. (1991). Reliability of retrospective assessments of sexual HIV risk behavior: A comparison of biweekly, three-month, and twelve-month self-reports. *AIDS Education and Prevention 3,* 207-214.

Kelly, J.A. (1997). HIV risk reduction interventions for persons with severe mental illness. *Clinical Psychology Review, 17,* 293-309.

Kelly, J. A., & Murphy, D. A. (1992). Psychological interventions with AIDS and HIV: Prevention and treatment. *Journal of Consulting and Clinical Psychology, 60,* 576-585.

Malow, R.M., Devieux, J., Martinez, L.M., Lucenko, B., & Kalichman, S.C. (in press). History of traumatic abuse and HIV risk behaviors in severely mentally ill substance abusing adults. *Journal of Family Violence.*

McKinnon, K., Cournos, F., Sugden, R., Guido, J.R., & Herman, R. (1996). The relative contribution of psychiatric symptoms and AIDS knowledge to HIV risk behaviors among people with severe mental illness. *Journal of Clinical Psychiatry, 57* (11), 506-573.

McKinnon, K., & Cournos, F. (1998). HIV infection linked to substance use among hospitalized patients with severe mental illness. *Psychiatric Services, 49,* 1269.

McLellan, A.T., Metzger, D., & Peters, R. (1992). The fifth edition of the Addiction Severity Index. *Journal of Substance Abuse Treatment, 9,* 207-214.

Miller, M. (1999). A model to explain the relationship between sexual abuse and HIV risk among women. *AIDS Care, 11*(1), 3-20.

Mueser, K. T., Goodman, L. B., & Trumbetta, S. L. (1998). Trauma and posttraumatic stress disorder in severe mental illness. *Journal of Consulting and Clinical Psychology 66,* 493-499.

Mueser, K.T., Rosenberg, S.D., Goodman, L.A., & Trumbetta, S.L. (2002). Trauma, PTSD, and the course of severe mental illness: An interactive model. *Schizophrenia Research, 53*(1-2), 123-143.

National Institute on Drug Abuse. (1991). *Risk behavior assessment.* Rockville, MD: National Institute on Drug Abuse.

Needle, R., Fisher, D., Weatherby, N., Brown, B., Cesari, H., Chitwood, D. et al. (1995). Reliability of self-reported HIV risk behaviors of drug users. *Psychology of Addictive Behaviors 9,* 242-250.

Otto-Salaj, L. L., Kelly, J. A., Stevenson, L.Y., Hoffman, R., & Kalichman, S. C. (2001). Outcomes of a randomized small group HIV prevention intervention trial for people with serious mental illness. *Community Mental Health Journal, 37,* 123-147.

RachBeisel, J., Scott, J., & Dixon, L. (1999). Co-occurring severe mental illness and substance use disorders: A review of recent research. *Psychiatric Services, 50,* 1427-1434.

Regier, D.A., Farmer, M.E., Rae, D.S., Locke, B.Z., Keith, S.J., Judd, L.L., & Goodwin, F.K. (1990). Co-morbidity of mental disorders with alcohol and other drug abuse. Results from the Epidemiological Catchment Area (ECA) study. *JAMA, 262,* 2511-2518.

Rosenberg, S.D., Drake, R.E., & Mueser, K.T. (1996). New directions for treatment research on sequelae of sexual abuse in persons with severe mental illness. *Community Mental Health Journal, 32,* 387-400.

Rosenberg, S.D., Goodman, L.A., Osher, F.C., Swartz, M.S., Essock, S.M., Butterfield, M. I. et al. (2001). Prevalence of HIV, Hepatitis B and Hepatitis C in people with severe mental illness. *American Journal of Public Health, 91,* 31-37.

Rosenberg, S.D., Mueser, K.T., Friedman, M.J., Gorman, P.G., Drake, R.E., Vidaver, R.M. et al. (2001). Developing effective treatments for posttraumatic disorders among people with severe mental illness. *Psychiatric Services, 52*(11), 1453-1461.

Zanis, D.A., McLellan, A.T., Cnaan, R.A., & Randall, M. (1994). Reliability and validity of the Addiction Severity Index with a homeless sample. *Journal of Substance Abuse Treatment, 11,*541-548.

doi:10.1300/J005v33n01_02

Symptom Cluster of Fatigue and Depression in HIV/AIDS

Joachim G. Voss

National Institutes of Health

Carmen J. Portillo
William L. Holzemer
Marylin J. Dodd

University of California San Francisco

SUMMARY. Fatigue and depression are among the most frequently rated symptoms of people with HIV/AIDS. This study aimed: (1) to describe severity of fatigue and depression in an outpatient sample (n = 372) of men and women with HIV/AIDS, (2) to evaluate sensitivity and discriminant validity for two fatigue and three depression scales and (3) to investigate whether fatigue and depression are conceptually distinct concepts or reciprocally dependent. This was a secondary analysis of a descriptive, cross-sectional study with convenience sampling. Fatigue was assessed with the fatigue factor score of the revised Sign and Symptom Checklist HIV (SSC-HIVrev), and the fatigue scale of the Self-Care Symptom Management for Living with HIV/AIDS Scale

---

Address correspondence to: Joachim G. Voss,, National Institutes of Health, National Institute of Neurological Disorders and Stroke, Neuromuscular Diseases Section, Building 10, Room 4N252, 10 Center Drive, MSC 1382, Bethesda, MD 20892-1382.

The authors give special thanks to Dr. Kathy Lee for her thoughtful review of this manuscript.

[Haworth co-indexing entry note]: "Symptom Cluster of Fatigue and Depression in HIV/AIDS." Voss, Joachim G. et al. Co-published simultaneously in *Journal of Prevention & Intervention in the Community* (The Haworth Press, Inc.) Vol. 33, No.1/2, 2007, pp. 19-34; and: *HIV: Issues with Mental Health and Illness* (ed: Michael B. Blank, and Marlene M. Eisenberg) The Haworth Press, Inc., 2007, pp. 19-34. Single or multiple copies of this article are available for a fee from The Haworth Document Delivery Service [1-800-HAWORTH, 9:00 a.m. - 5:00 p.m. (EST). E-mail address: docdelivery@ haworthpress.com].

(SCSMS-F). Depression was assessed with the depression factor score of the SSC-HIVrev, the depression scale of the SCSMC-D and the Center for Epidemiologic Studies Depression Scale (CES-D). Most of the participants were male (67%), with a mean age of 39.9 years, and of African American decent (73%). Dependent on the instrument, the average fatigue severity was moderate and the average depression severity was moderate to severe. Women experienced higher fatigue and depression severity scores than men. The scores on the same instruments for fatigue and depression showed significant correlations (SSC-HIVrev fatigue and depression $r = 0.62$; SCSMS fatigue and depression $r = 0.64$), indicating that both concepts are closely related. Patients seeking help for fatigue and/or depression should always be evaluated for both symptoms. Future research is needed to identify dimensions in different fatigue and depression scales in order to differentiate the impact of both symptoms on people living with HIV/AIDS. doi:10.1300/J005v33n01_03   *[Article copies available for a fee from The Haworth Document Delivery Service: 1-800-HAWORTH. E-mail address: <docdelivery@haworthpress.com> Website: <http://www.HaworthPress.com> © 2007 by The Haworth Press, Inc. All rights reserved.]*

KEYWORDS. Fatigue, depression, measurement assessment, African-American

Symptom clusters for two or more symptoms are groups of symptoms, where one symptom overlaps or mimics secondary symptoms. The major challenge is to identify the presence of either symptom to assure correct diagnosis and treatment. Fatigue and depression assessment relies solely on subjective ratings by the patient and the provider. This subjective assessment leaves a wide possibility for introducing diagnostic and treatment bias, by the patient dependent on literacy, culture, or adjustment to the symptom severity, and by the provider in terms of knowledge, priorities, and willingness for ongoing assessment. The following article will provide a brief review about fatigue and depression and describe the study findings of a group of HIV/AIDS outpatients from Texas. The main focus will be methodological issues and recommendations in terms of evaluation of fatigue and depression.

FATIGUE

Fatigue in HIV/AIDS has been reported to cause depression, limit quality of life, and decrease cognitive, physical and social functioning

(Barroso et al., 2002; Breitbart, Rosenfeld, Kaim, & Funesti-Esch, 2001). In addition, fatigue is considered to be one of the primary symptoms of a clinical depression (Perkins et al., 1995). Fatigue is the most prevalent and debilitating symptom in people with HIV/AIDS and prevalence rates of up to 85% have been reported (Lee, Portillo & Miramontes, 1999; Sullivan & Dworkin, 2003; Vogl et al., 1999). Fatigue limits patients' functional and psychological abilities, and decreases the ability to work and to maintain social relationships (Barroso, 1999; Cunningham et al., 1998). Due to the high prevalence of fatigue and depression in HIV/AIDS patients, major attempts have been made to separate the two concepts into single entities with little success (Breitbart et al., 2001; Wagner & Rabkin, 2000).

Chronic fatigue in HIV/AIDS is defined as a permanent physical and/ or mental exhaustion and tiredness that persists for longer than one month (Piper et al., 1998). It is independent of the amount of rest and sleep and often worsens with increasing hours of sleep, also known as secondary fatigue (Winningham et al., 1994). The development of fatigue is multifactorial, and for a review see (Barroso, 1999), and while progress has been made in understanding the underlying patho-physiology of fatigue, there is still a wide gap in the objective assessment and diagnosis of this widespread symptom.

Fatigue is a subjective perception of the patient, usually rated on numeric (0-10) or Likert scales (mild–moderate–severe), mostly assessing the presence, severity, and impact of fatigue. Attempts to correlate fatigue to objective measures such as CD4 + T cell count, viral load, or hemoglobin (Barroso, Carlson, & Meynell, 2003) have failed so far. Similar to the assessment of fatigue, the diagnosis currently relies on the subjective judgment of healthcare providers. Dependent on the experience level of the healthcare provider to recognize fatigue as a significant problem, patients' symptom experiences possibly translate into diagnosis and treatment. Equally to HIV/AIDS patients, cancer patients report similar high prevalence rates for fatigue (Mock & Olsen, 2003), indicating an urgent need to develop valid and reliable diagnostic criteria. Cella and colleagues (1998) drafted diagnostic criteria for cancer-related fatigue in order to establish an independent ICD-10 code (International Classification of Diseases, WHO, 1992) (Cella et al., 1998). However, these diagnostic criteria have never been systematically investigated nor found acceptance across healthcare professionals for the diagnosis of cancer-related fatigue. Despite the standardization issue, these criteria could readily be applied to the assessment and diagnosis of HIV/AIDS-related fatigue. The four diagnostic criteria include the presence of six or more symptoms related to fatigue, that symptoms contribute to clinically significant distress or impairment, that symptoms are sequelae of cancer or cancer therapy (possibly changed to HIV/AIDS and HIV therapy), and that the symptoms are not primarily a consequence of comorbid psychiatric conditions such as major depression. The symptoms associated with the criteria include significant fatigue, general weakness or limb heaviness, diminished concentration, decreased motivation, insomnia or hypersomnia, experience of non-restorative sleep, perceived struggle to overcome inactivity, marked emotional reactivity to feeling fatigued (e.g., sadness, frustration, or irritability), difficulty completing daily tasks attributable to feeling fatigued, perceived problems with short-term memory, and malaise post-exertion lasting several hours (Cella et al., 1998). These diagnostic criteria attempt to separate depression from fatigue as a primary diagnosis, considering that fatigue affects mood.

DEPRESSION

The lifetime risk of developing clinical depression without HIV is 7% to 12% for men and 20% to 25% for women. Risk factors for men and women include: post-partum depression, history of depressive illness in first-degree relatives, prior episodes of major depression, prior suicide attempts, being over 40 years of age, medical comorbidity, decreased social support, stressful life events, and current substance or alcohol abuse (NIMH, 2002; Weissman et al., 1996). Prevalence rates of depression for people with HIV/AIDS have been reported as high as 50%, especially in women, African-Americans, homeless, and drug-using populations (Bing et al., 2001; Low-Beer et al., 2000; Cruess et al., 2003). The development of depression with HIV disease is also multidimensional (for review see Dean et al., 2004; Leserman, 2004). In addition, treatments for HIV disease such as Efavirenz may trigger the onset of a major depression (Puzantian, 2002).

The complex pathophysiological nature of depression complicates the diagnostic process by presenting the disease through multiple symptoms and limitations, including affective, somatic, cognitive, and behavioral changes. These difficulties in diagnosing depression are reflected in the four major existing diagnostic approaches. Dependent on inclusion or exclusion of physical symptoms as diagnostic criteria four major approaches are utilized to diagnose depression: (1) the inclusive approach by Rifkin and colleagues (1985) where all symptoms are counted in making a diagnosis of depression whether or not they may be attributable to a physical problem (Rifkin et al., 1985); (2) the etiological approach by Spitzer and Wakefield (1999), developer of the Diagnostic and Statistical Manual of Mental Disorders (DSM), which requires an interviewer to attribute causal somatic symptoms to depression. Sleep disturbances, appetite disturbances, fatigue, psychomotor agitation or retardation, and changes in concentration can only be counted towards a diagnosis with depression if they are not clearly due to a physical illness; (3) the exclusive approach by Roth and colleagues (1998), which simply eliminates fatigue and appetite disturbances from the diagnostic criteria, in order to keep the diagnostic process free from somatic symptoms (Roth et al., 1998); and (4) the substitutive approach by Endicott (1984), which replaces somatic symptoms of depression with affective symptoms. For example, appetite disturbances were replaced with fearfulness or depressed appearance; and fatigue with brooding, self-pity or pessimism (Endicott, 1984).

Studies that focused exclusively on affective/cognitive symptoms of depression appeared to be more discriminatory than focusing on somatic/vegetative symptoms (Jones, Beach, & Forehand, 2001; Kalechstein, Hinkin, van Gorp, Castellon, & Satz, 1998; Penzak, Reddy, & Grimsley, 2000). Jones and colleagues (2001) conducted a longitudinal study to assess the risk for depressive symptoms among HIV-infected African American single mothers (n = 96), relative to demographically matched healthy single mothers (n = 120). They used the self-report depression sub-scale of the brief symptom inventory (BSI), and the clinician-rated Hamilton Rating Scale for Depression (HRSD). Depressive symptoms were assessed at the onset of the study and after 12 months. Findings revealed that HIV-infected mothers were at greater risk for depressive symptoms at both assessments, regardless of method of assessment. BSI scores were significantly higher for HIV infected mothers after 12 month, compared to the non-infected mothers. Moreover, HIV-infected mothers remained at greater risk when the analyses were limited to cognitive and affective symptoms of depression. This decreased the likelihood that the difference between the two groups was due to greater endorsement of somatic symptoms of depression by the HIV-infected group.

In summary, both symptoms are highly prevalent in HIV/AIDS patients and affect patients physically, mentally, psychologically, and socially. Considering the previous findings in fatigue and depression research, the major question is: should both concepts always be investigated jointly to capture their overlapping effects, and if not, can they be investigated separately?

The purpose of this study was to demonstrate the level of fatigue and depression in a sample of men and women with HIV/AIDS and to investigate methodological issues for both symptoms. Therefore, we proposed three aims: (1) Evaluate the prevalence of fatigue and depression in a sample of men and women with HIV/AIDS with different symptom assessment and depression tools; (2) evaluate the sensitivity and discriminant validity of two fatigue and three depression scales; and (3) investigate whether fatigue and depression are distinct concepts or should be considered reciprocally dependent.

METHODS

Design/Setting/Sample

This was a descriptive, correlational, secondary data analysis. The original study was conducted at a large urban HIV outpatient clinic in Texas, which served approximately 5,200 HIV/AIDS clients. Within a three week period, all patients scheduled for their regular appointments were given the opportunity to participate in the study. Out of the 384 patients that came to the clinic during this period, a convenience sample of 372 HIV/AIDS patients completed the questionnaire booklet. The original study focused on the psychometric analysis of a symptom assessment instrument for people with HIV/AIDS. The participants received $10 for their participation, which took approximately 45 minutes to complete.

Instruments

For this study, a questionnaire booklet included the following self-report instruments: demographic data set, the revised Sign and Symptom Checklist HIV (SSC-HIVrev), the Self-Care Symptom Management Scale for People Living with HIV/AIDS (SCSMS), and the Center for Epidemiologic Studies Depression Scale (CES-D). A brief introduction of each scale will be following:

The SSC-HIVrev is a self-report 74-item list of the most common signs and symptoms in HIV/AIDS disease, eight of which are gynecological. Severity and frequency of each symptom are assessed with an ordinal three-point Likert scale (mild, moderate, and severe). The four-item factor cluster for fatigue (fatigue, muscle aches, painful joints, and weakness) and the four-item factor cluster for depression (difficulty concentrating, depression, memory loss, and fear) (Holzemer et al., 1999;

Holzemer et al., 2001) were evaluated for their reliability coefficient. The analysis revealed strong reliability coefficients for each item of the fatigue ($\alpha = 0.86$) and the depression ($\alpha = 0.87$) factor scores.

The SCSMS is an instrument that was utilized first in a web-based study to investigate self-care management of HIV symptoms (www. hivsymptoms.com). In this study patients were asked to rate any of the following six symptoms by presence in the last week (1-7 days), intensity (1-10), bothersomeness (1-10), and the degree to which it affected their daily lives (1-10): (1) anxiety/fear, (2) nausea/vomiting, (3) depression, (4) neuropathy, (5) fatigue, and (6) diarrhea. For this analysis, the two scales for fatigue and depression were included. Cronbach's α was calculated for both scales and reached ($\alpha = 0.92$) for the fatigue scale and ($\alpha = 0.90$) for the depression scale indicating a strong coherence between the items.

The CES-D is a well-established, 20-item scale, utilized as a standardized, self-report, non-diagnostic screening tool for depressive symptoms, which measures depressive symptoms within community populations (Radloff, 1977). For the men and women (N = 275) with HIV/AIDS that completed the CES-D in this sample, Cronbach's α reached ($\alpha = 0.88$), indicating an excellent reliability among all items and confirming previous findings that this scale is reliable in measuring depressive symptoms in HIV/AIDS samples.

RESULTS

Sociodemographic and HIV Characteristics of the Sample

The following results will represent all participants that completed either the demographic information or the symptom scales or both. We did not substitute missing values with the mean for any missing data; therefore, each analysis has different total numbers. The mean age was 39.9 years (±8.3, range 18-66). Most participants were men (68%). Of the total sample, there were 271 (73%) African Americans, 55 (15%) Caucasians, 33 (9%) Latinos, and 13 (4%) were of diverse ethnic background. African Americans were disproportionately higher represented than in the U.S. average African American HIV/AIDS cases, which is 50%. A large proportion of the participants (59%) lacked sufficient education and did not finish high school. Almost 70% of the men and women considered themselves as disabled, and 56.7% reported an inadequate income. Only 29%

stated that their health insurance was sufficient to cover their healthcare needs, and the majority of the participants were unemployed (85%).

The year HIV infection occurred was unknown to 53% of the participants. Of those who identified the year of HIV infection, 7.3% were infected between 1982-1990, and 39.7% between 1991-2000. Knowledge of the year of AIDS diagnosis differed greatly from the time of HIV infection; 91.6% of the respondents reported their current AIDS status, of which 54% identified themselves as having AIDS. The mean CD4 + T cell count, known by 42%, was 452/mm³ (± 315/mm³, range 2-1800/ mm³ CD4+ T cells). Viral load values were known by 42%, with a mean of 44,893 copies (± 166,688, range 0-1 million viral copies).

Severity of Fatigue and Depression in Men and Women with HIV/AIDS

In order to evaluate the prevalence of fatigue, only scores that reached the moderate to severe level were considered as truly fatigued and not as a naturally occurring tiredness due to daily variations of energy levels. When the scores of the SSC-HIVrev fatigue score (4 and above) and the SCSMS fatigue score (14 and above) reached 33% or above, patients were considered chronically fatigued. For the SSC-HIVrev fatigue score, 71% of the sample reported moderate to severe fatigue. For the SCSMS fatigue scale, 77% of the participants scored 14 and above. The mean fatigue score for the SSC-HIVrev fatigue factor scale was moderate 5.7 (± 3.6, range 1-12), and moderate 22.0 (± 10.1, range 1-37) for the SCSMS fatigue scale. To assess the differences in fatigue severity by gender and age, t-tests and ANOVAs were calculated. Women reported higher SSC-HIVrev fatigue mean scores than men 6.3 (± 3.7, range 1-12) vs. 5.4 (± 3.7, range 1-12, t = 2.11, p < 0.035). The differences for the SCSMS fatigue scores (women = 21.5/men = 22.6) were not significantly different. To evaluate fatigue in terms of age, three age groups were created according to previous findings in people with HIV/AIDS (Singh, 1997; Trotta et al., 2003; Zingmond et al., 2003). Group one (n = 32) ranged from 18-29 called ("Young"), group two (n = 284) from 30-49 ("Middle Age"), and group three (n = 46) from 50-66 ("Older"). The highest SSC-HIVrev fatigue scores were reported by the Middle Age group with 5.8 (± 3.6), the lowest by the Young group (5.0 ± 3.7), but the differences were not significant (F = 0.992, p = 0.372). The highest SCSMS fatigue score was reported by the Young group (n = 11) (24.6 ± 12), the lowest by the Older group (n = 18) (20.2 ± 8.0), yet not significantly different (F = 0.671, p = 0.513).

Similar to the fatigue measures, we considered depression as clinically relevant beyond 33% of the SSC-HIVrev depression factor score and the SCSMS-depression scale. The CES-D has a standardized cut-off of 16 as an indicator to screen for the presence of clinical depression. For the SSC-HIVrev depression score, 71% of the sample reported moderate to severe depression. For the SCSMS-depression scale, 79% of the participants scored 14 and above. For the CES-D, 87.6% scored above 16, indicating a high prevalence of moderate to severe depression. The mean depression score for the SSC-HIVrev depression factor scale was 5.5 (± 3.6, range 1-12) and 22.3 (± 9.3, range 1-37) for the SCSMS depression scale. The number of depressive symptoms for the CES-D was high with an average of 28.1 symptoms (±11.1, range 0-60). To investigate the differences of depression scores by gender and age, t-tests and ANOVAs were calculated. Women reported in general, higher mean scores on depression on the SSC-HIVrev depression scale (6.2 ± 3.7, range 1-12) than did men (5.2 ± 3.6, range 1-12), t = 2.261, p < 0.024). On the CES-D, women reported significantly more depressive symptoms than men, [women (30.1 ± 12.5) versus men 27.2 (±10.2), t = 02.36, p < 0.01]. Similar to the SCSMS fatigue ratings, the differences for the SCSMS depression scores between men and women (women = 21.7/men = 23.3) were not significantly different. To evaluate depression in terms of age, the same three age groups were created as for fatigue. Equally high SSC-HIVrev depression scores were reported by the Young (n = 32) and the Middle Age group (n = 284) (5.7 ± 3.5/3.7), the lowest by the Older group (n = 46) (4.7 ± 3.5), but the differences were not significant (F = 1.460, p = 0.234). The highest SCSMS depression score was reported by the Middle Age group (22.4 ± 9.4), the lowest by the Young group (20.8 ± 12.1), but the differences were not significantly different (F = 0.175, p = 0.840). The highest CES-D depression score was reported by the Young group (n = 32) (30.3 ± 11.2) and the Middle Age group (n = 284) (28.8 ± 10.8), but the differences were not significant. The lowest score was found in the Older group (n = 46) (22.3 ± 11.3), which was significantly different from the Younger and the Middle Age group (F = 7.659, p < 0.001).

Sensitivity and Validity of Fatigue and Depression Scales

Sensitivity and validity of two fatigue and three depression scales was evaluated to distinguish between fatigued and non-fatigued and depressed versus non-depressed patients. Subject who scored below 33% on each scale were considered not fatigued or not depressed. Their ratings were seen as an expression of natural daily changes in mood and energy, therefore clinically not significant. In the absence of a true control group, they became the control group against which we assessed the differences in the truly fatigued/depressed group in all five scales. The means and standard deviations for all patients and controls were significantly different for all five scales: SSC-Fatigue 2.1 ± 1.6 versus 8.3 ± 2.1 (p < 0.01); SCSMS Fatigue 8.6 ± 2.7 versus 29.9 ± 7.8 (p < 0.01); SSC-Depression 2.0 ± 1.6 versus 8.2 ± 2.2 (p < 0.01); SCSMS-Depression 9.3 ± 3.3 versus 25.6 ± 7.2 (p < 0.01); CES-D 10.2 ± 5.0 versus 30.6 ± 9.2 (p < 0.01). For the CES-D, which was the only standardized tool, we compared the mean scores of each item between the depressed and control group items. Significant differences for 18 of the 20 CES-D items were found (data not shown). Items which did not show significant differences between the depressed and control patients were "happy" and "enjoy life." To evaluate the discriminant validity of two fatigue and three depression scales, three correlation matrixes evaluated the scale correlations within the same and between the different concepts (see Tables 1-3). The correlation coefficient between the SSC-HIVrev and the SCSMS fatigue measure was highly significant at $r = 0.43$ (see Table 1). The coefficients for the SSC-HIVrev depression and the SCSMS depression scores were significantly correlated at $r = 0.63$, as well as for the SSC-HIVrev depression and the CES-D score at $r = 0.49$, and were correlated for the SCSMS depression and the CES-D score at $r = 0.45$ (see Table 2). All correlations between the fatigue and depression measures were significant at $p < 0.01$ (see Table 3). The correlation for the SSC-HIVrev fatigue score and the SSC-HIVrev depression score was $r = 0.63$, the SSC-HIVrev fatigue and the SCSMS depression score was $r = 0.42$, and the SSC-HIVrev fatigue and the CES-D score was $r = 0.33$. The correlation for the SCSMS fatigue score and SCSMS depression score was the highest at $r = 0.64$, and the lowest for the SCSMS fatigue score and the CES-D at $r = 0.28$.

Fatigue and Depression–Two Sides of the Same Coin

We analyzed whether fatigue and depression should be investigated separately or together. Three questions were asked whether there is a relationship between severity of depressive symptoms and fatigue, which we tried to answer with ANOVAs: (1) Do HIV/AIDS patients report non to

TABLE 1. Correlation Coefficient Matrix for Two Fatigue Measures

Instrument	SSCrev-Fatigue	SCSMS Fatigue	Mean Correlation
SSCrev-Fatigue	1.0	0.43*	0.43
SCSMS Fatigue		1.0	0.43

* Correlation is significant at the 0.01 level (two-tailed)

TABLE 2. Correlation Coefficient Matrix for Three Depression Measures

Instrument	SSCrev-Depression	SCSMS Depression	CES-D	Mean Correlation
SSCrev-Depression	1.0	0.63*	0.49**	0.56
SCSMS Depression		1.0	0.45	0.45
CES-D			1.0	0.51

* Correlation is significant at the 0.01 level (two-tailed)
** Correlation is significant at the 0.001 level (two-tailed)

TABLE 3. Correlation Coefficient Matrix for Two Fatigue and Three Depression Measures

Instrument	SSCrev-Fatigue	SCSMS Fatigue	SSCrev-Depression	SCSMS Depression	CES-D
SSCrev-Fatigue	1.0	0.43*	0.63*	0.42*	0.33*
SCSMS Fatigue		1.0	0.48*	0.64*	0.28*
SSCrev-Depression			1.0	0.57*	0.49*
SCSMS Depression				1.0	0.45*
CES-D					1.0

* Correlation is significant at the 0.01 level (two-tailed)

low fatigue severity with a CES-D score less than 16?; (2) Do HIV/AIDS patients report mild to moderate fatigue severity with a CES-D score between 16 and 22?; and (3) Do HIV/AIDS patients report high fatigue severity with a CES-D score above 23? If fatigue and depression are as closely related conceptually as expected, then there would be a positive relationship between increasing CES-D scores and increasing fatigue scores. The cut-off points were selected according to previous findings, where the authors suggested that the recommended cut-off point of 16 may be too low for African Americans (Lyon & Munro, 2001; Schulberg et al., 1985; Thomason, Jones, McClure & Mertens, 1997). Therefore, two cut-off points were chosen at 16 and 23. Of those who completed the CES-D and the fatigue scale of the HIV-SSCrev, 44 subjects with a CES-D score below 16, had a mean SSC-HIVrev fatigue factor score of 3.9 ($\pm$ 3.2). There were 78 subjects with a CES-D score between 16 and 23 and a fatigue score of 5.1, while 242 had a CES-D score higher than 23 with a fatigue score of 6.3. The differences between the three groups were assessed with ANOVA. Groups one and two were not significantly different, however, the comparisons between group one and three, and group two and three were significant different, ($F = 10.494$, $p < 0.001$), supporting the conclusion that there is a rise in the number of depressive symptoms with increasing fatigue severity.

DISCUSSION

We investigated the severity of fatigue and depression in a community sample of HIV/AIDS outpatients, and evaluated sensitivity and discriminant validity for two fatigue and three depression scales. Our findings confirm previous findings where people with HIV/AIDS suffer greatly from this debilitating symptom (Barroso, 1999; Breitbart et al., 2001; Cunningham et al., 1998). Furthermore, more than 3/4 of the participants qualified for an evaluation for major depression according to the cut-off point of 16 for the CES-D. This high number of depressive symptoms within participants of a single study is yet unexplained. Previous investigators found equally high numbers of depressive symptoms, especially in African American samples (Hudson, Kirksey, & Holzemer, 2004; Jones, Beach, Forehand, & Foster, 2003; Lyons & Murno, 2001), and the authors agree with previous investigators that 16 as the cut-off point may be too low. Future studies would need to determine a more appropriate cut-off point.

The investigation about conceptual distinct differences between fatigue and depression revealed that with increasing depression, patients become increasingly fatigued, supporting the conclusion that both symptoms should always be evaluated jointly. All scales for fatigue and depression were sensitive enough to capture the symptom experience of participants in order to distinguish between those that were fatigued and non-fatigued or depressed or non-depressed. However, the scales did not provide evidence for discriminant validity indicating a significant conceptual overlap between fatigue and depression and the need for joint assessment. While there is an ongoing debate of physical versus affective symptoms to evaluate depression, one would expect a clear distinction between the fatigue and depression factor score of the SSC-HIVrev. Each factor score included either somatic (fatigue) or affective (depression) symptoms, yet the correlation coefficient between both factor scores was high at $r = 0.62$. This indicates that evaluating patients with symptom scales may be sensitive enough to evaluate for symptoms, yet not specific enough to establish a final diagnosis.

Similar to the SSC-HIVrev, both scales of the SCSMS identified between 77% to 80% of people with fatigue and depression and confirmed the scales sensitivity to identify those with moderate to severe symptoms. These findings confirmed that the four-item scales were sufficient to identify participants with fatigue or depression and provide precise information about the symptom experience of people living with HIV/AIDS. However, a correlation of 0.64 indicates a lack in specificity for a final diagnosis of fatigue or depression and more specific data is needed to further validate the scales.

Limitations of this study were a lack of including a multidimensional fatigue scale and the lack of a control group. Also, the symptom reports were acquired by self-report and not confirmed by clinical evaluation. In the future, qualitative research for depressed and non-depressed African American HIV/AIDS patients may provide insights into the reasons for higher depression scores on the CES-D in this group than in any other ethnic group.

CONCLUSIONS

Diagnosis for depression or fatigue is difficult and requires the full attention of healthcare providers and open discussions between patients and providers. Both symptoms occur as a cluster, are closely related, and need to be monitored throughout the course of the HIV disease in order to avoid decreases in quality of life. Measures of fatigue and depression should be multi-dimensional to understand the impact both symptoms have on the individual in order to make appropriate recommendations for interventions. Ethnic-specific research is needed to elaborate on our findings and detect the differences in language, culture, and symptom representation in African Americans. Especially, African Americans living with HIV/AIDS need to be screened for depression and fatigue to assure adequate treatment. More research is needed to understand the complex interplay between fatigue and depression with new collaborative approaches.

REFERENCES

Barroso, J. (1999). A review of fatigue in people with HIV infection. *Journal of the Association of Nurses in AIDS Care, 10*(5), 42-9.

Barroso, J., Carlson, J.R., & Meynell, J. (2003). Physiological and psychological markers associated with HIV-related fatigue. *Clinical Nursing Research, 12*(1), 49-68.

Barroso, J., Preisser, J. S., Leserman, J., Gaynes, B. N., Golden, R. N., & Evans, D. N. (2002). Predicting fatigue and depression in HIV-positive men. *Psychosomatics, 43*(4), 317-25.

Bing, E. G., Burnam, M. A., Longshore, D., Fleishman, J. A., Sherbourne, C. D., London, A. S., Turner, B. J., Eggan, F. et al. (2001). Psychiatric disorders and drug use among human immunodeficiency virus-infected adults in the United States. *Archives of General Psychiatry, 58*(8), 721-8.

Breitbart, W., Rosenfeld, B., Kaim, M., & Funesti-Esch, J. (2001). A randomized, double-blind, placebo-controlled trial of psychostimulants for the treatment of fatigue in ambulatory patients with human immunodeficiency virus disease. *Archives of Internal Medicine, 161*(3), 411-20.

Cella, D., Peterman, A., Passik, S., Jacobson, P., & Breitbart, W. (1998). Progress towards guidelines for the management of fatigue. *Oncology, 12*(11), 369-77.

Cruess, D. G., Dwight, L. E., Repetto, M. J., Gettes, D., Douglas, S. D., & Petitto, D. (2003). Prevalence, diagnosis, and pharmacological treatment of mood disorders in HIV disease. *Biological Psychiatry, 54*, 307-316.

Cunningham, W. E., Shapiro, M. F., Hays, R. D., Dixon, W. J., Visscher, B. R., George, W. L., Ettl, M. K., & Beck, C. K. (1998). Constitutional symptoms and health-related quality of life in patients with symptomatic HIV disease. *American Journal of Medicine, 104*(2), 129-36.

Endicott, J. (1984). Measurement of depression in patients with cancer. *Cancer; 53*, 2243-48.

Hudson, A., Kirksey, K., & Holzemer, W. (2004). The influences of symptoms on quality of life among HIV-infected women. *Western Journal of Nursing Research, 26*(1), 9-23.

Jones, D. J., Beach, S. R., Forehand, R., & Foster, S. E. (2003). Self-reported health in HIV-positive African American women: The role of family stress and depressive symptoms. *Journal of Behavioral Medicine,26*(6), 577-99.

Lee, K. A., Portillo, C. J., & Miramontes, H. (1999). The fatigue experience for women with human immunodeficiency virus. *Journal of Obstetric, Gynecologic, and Neonatal Nursing, 28*(2), 193-200.

Low-Beer, S., Chan, K., Yip, B., Wood, E., Montaner, J. S., O'Shaughnessy, M. V. & Hogg, R. S. (2000). Depressive symptoms decline among persons with HIV protease inhibitors. *Journal of Acquired Immune Deficiency Syndromes, 23*, 295-301.

Lyons, D. E. & Munro, C. (2001). Disease severity and symptoms of depression in black Americans infected with HIV. *Applied Nursing Research, 14*(1), 3-10.

Mock, V. & Olson, M. (2003). Current management of fatigue and anemia in patients with cancer. *Seminars of Oncology Nursing, 19*(4 Suppl 2), 36-41.

National Institute of Mental Health. Depression. Bethesda (MD): National Institute of Mental Health, National Institutes of Health, US Department of Health and Human Services; 2000 [reprinted 2002; cited 2004 January 26]. (NIH Publication Number: NIH 02-3561). 23 pages. Available from: http://www.nimh.nih.gov/publicat/depression.cfm

Perkins, D. O., Leserman, J., Stern, R. A., Baum, S. F., Liao, D., Golden, R. N., & Evans, D. L. (1995). Somatic symptoms and HIV infection: Relationship to depressive symptoms and indicators of HIV disease. *American Journal of Psychiatry, 152*(12), 1776-81.

Piper, B. (1998). Fatigue. In M. E. Ropka (Ed.), *HIV nursing and symptom management*. Boston: Jones and Bartlett.

Puzantian, T. (2002). Central nervous system adverse effects with efavirenz: Case report and review. *Pharmacotherapy, 22*(7), 930-3.

Salomon, J., de Truchis, P., & Melchoir, J. C. (2002). Body composition and nutritional parameters in HIV and AIDS patients. *Clinical Chemistry and Laboratory Medicine, 40*(12), 1329-33.

Schulberg, H. C., Saul, M., & McClelland, M. (1985). Assessing depression in primary medical and psychiatric practices. *Archives of General Psychiatry, 42*(12), 1164-70.

Spitzer, R. L., & Wakefield, J. C. (1999). DSM-IV diagnostic criterion for clinical significance: Does it help solve the false positives problem? *American Journal of Psychiatry, 156*(12), 1856-64.

Sullivan, P. S. & Dworkin, M. S.; Adult and Adolescent Spectrum of HIV Diseases Investigators. (2003). Prevalence and correlates of fatigue among persons with HIV Infection. *Journal of Pain and Symptom Management; 25*(4), 329-33.

Thomason, B., Jones, G., McClure, J., & Brantley, P. (1996). Psychosocial co-factors in HIV illness: An empirically-based model. *Psychology and Health,11*, 385-93.

Vogl, D., Rosenfeld, B., Breitbart, W., Thaler, H., Passik, S., McDonald, M., & Portenoy, R. K. (1999). Symptom prevalence, characteristics, and distress in AIDS outpatients. *Journal of Pain and Symptom Management, 18*(4), 253-62.

Wagner, G. J., & Rabkin, R. (2000). Effects of dextroamphetamine on depression and fatigue in men with HIV: A double-blind, placebo-controlled trial. *Journal of Clinical Psychiatry, 61*(6), 436-40.

Weissman, M. M., Bland, R. C., Canino, G. J., Faravelli, C., Greenwald, S., Hwu, H. G., Joyce, P. R., Karam, E. G., Lee, C. K., Lellouch, J., Lepine, J. P., Newman, S. C., Rubin-Stiper, M., Wells, J. E., Wickramaratne, P. J., Wittchen, H., & Yeh, E. K.

(1996). Cross-national epidemiology of major depression and bipolar disorder. *Journal of the American Medical Association, 276,* 293-99.

Winningham, M. L., Nail, L. M., Burke, M. B., Brophy, L., Cimprich, B., Jones, L. S., Pickard Holley, S., Rhodes, V., St Pierre, B., Beck, S., Glass, E. C., Mock, V. L., Mooney, K. H., & Piper, B. (1994). Fatigue and the cancer experience: The state of the knowledge. *Oncology-Nursing-Forum, 21*(1), 23-36.

World Health Organization. (1992). *International Diagnostic Classification (ICD-10).* Geneva: World Health Organization. Available: http://www.who.int/msa/mnh/ems/icd10/cliexamp.htm [2001, July 1].

doi:10.1300/J005v33n01_03

Emotional Distress
in African American Women with HIV

Margaret Shandor Miles
Diane Holditch-Davis
Cort Pedersen
Joseph J.Eron, Jr.
Todd Schwartz

The University of North Carolina at Chapel Hill

SUMMARY. This study identified factors associated with emotional distress in 109 African American women with HIV. The relationship of personal factors (demographic, social conflict, social support, and spirituality), health-related factors (perception of health, physical and mental health problems, and years diagnosed), and cognitive/coping responses (stigma, worry, and emotion focused coping) on depressive symptoms

---

Address correspondence to: Margaret Shandor Miles, 530 Carrington Hall CB 7460, Chapel Hill, NC 27599-7460 (E-mail: mmiles@email.unc.edu).

The authors wish to acknowledge the staff who assisted in this project, particularly Beth Perry Black, MSN, Project Director and Donna Harris, BSN; Jenise V. Gillespie, RN, PhD, Valerie Lunsford, MSN; and Hyekyun Rhee, PhD.

Funding for this study was provided by the National Institute of Nursing Research, National Institutes of Health (R01 NR04416). Partial support also came from NIH funded centers: The Center for AIDS Research (P30 AI50410), the General Clinical Research Center (RR00046), and the Center for Research on Chronic Illness (P30 NR 03962) awarded to the Schools of Medicine and Nursing at the University of North Carolina at Chapel Hill.

[Haworth co-indexing entry note]: "Emotional Distress in African American Women with HIV." Miles, Margaret Shandor et al. Co-published simultaneously in *Journal of Prevention & Intervention in the Community* (The Haworth Press, Inc.) Vol. 33, No.1/2, 2007, pp. 35-50; and: *HIV: Issues with Mental Health and Illness* (ed: Michael B. Blank, and Marlene M. Eisenberg) The Haworth Press, Inc., 2007, pp. 35-50. Single or multiple copies of this article are available for a fee from The Haworth Document Delivery Service [1-800-HAWORTH, 9:00 a.m. - 5:00 p.m. (EST). E-mail address: docdelivery@ haworthpress.com].

Available online at http://jpic.haworthpress.com
doi:10.1300/J005v33n01_04

and mood state was examined. Younger age, more social conflict, less social support, lower perception of health, and more HIV worry were associated with higher depressive symptom scores. Variables most often affecting various mood states included personal factors (public housing, unemployment, and social conflict) and worry about having HIV worry.

doi:10.1300/J005v33n01_04 *[Article copies available for a fee from The Haworth Document Delivery Service: 1-800-HAWORTH. E-mail address: <docdelivery@ haworthpress.com> Website: <http://www.HaworthPress.com>* © 2007 by The Haworth Press, Inc. All rights reserved.]*

KEYWORDS. African American women, HIV, emotional distress

There is increasing evidence of psychological distress and mental health problems among individuals with HIV (Bing et al., 2001; Ciesla & Roberts, 2001; Orlando et al., 2002). Women with HIV are especially at risk for psychological distress, particularly depression (Catz, Gore-Felton, & McClure, 2002; Cook et al., 2004; Kaplan, Marks, & Mertens, 1997; Mellins, Kang, Leu, Havens, & Chesney, 2003; Miles, Burchinal, Holditch-Davis, Wasilewszki, & Christian, 1996; Moneyham, Sowell, Seals, & Demi, 2000; Morrison et al., 2002). Identifying the factors associated with emotional distress and mental health problems in women with HIV is an important step towards developing interventions to improve mental health. The most salient factors appear to be related to personal and family characteristics. Numerous studies found lower social support associated with poorer mental health or more emotional distress (Catz et al., 2002; Fleishman et al., 2000; Gielen, McDonnell, Wu, O'Campo, & Faden, 2001; Hudson et al., 2001; Lapedagne, Ferriere, Lacoste, & Verdoux, 2000; Mellins et al., 2003; Pakenham & Rinaldis, 2001; Serovich, Kimerly, Mosack, & Lewis, 2001; Silver, Bauman, Camacho, & Hudis, 2003). Too, unsupportive relationships with family and others are associated with depression (Fleishman et al., 2000; Schrimshaw, 2003). Spirituality has also been associated with well-being for African Americans (Coleman & Holzemer, 1999) and factors associated with poverty, such as unemployment and socioeconomic status, have been implicated in depression (Blalock, McDaniel, & Farber, 2002; Bing et al., 2001).

A variety of health-related factors have also been associated with psychological distress in individuals with HIV. Ciesla and Roberts (2001), based on their meta-analysis, concluded that rates of depression are not related to disease stage of infected individuals. However, emotional distress and depression may be higher in the period following diagnosis (Ciesla & Roberts, 2001; Lapedagne et al., 2000). HIV-related symptoms, health quality of life, and other health problems were associated with depression in several studies (Bing et al., 2001; Heckman et al., 2004; Miles et al., 1997; Moneyham et al., 2000; Pakenham & Rinaldis, 2001; Silver et al., 2003; Tostes, Chalub, & Botega, 2004).

Limited attention has been placed on how one's response to having HIV relates to emotional distress. HIV-related stigma was a predictor of depressive symptoms in African American women (Miles et al., 1997). Postpartum women with HIV in Thailand reported high levels of worry, but the relationship between worry and depression was not examined (Bennetts et al., 1999). Franke, Jager, Thomann, and Beyer (1992) reported that worry and isolation were salient characteristics of German women with psychological distress. However, worry was not systematically measured in either study. Several studies examined the impact of coping strategies on distress. Problem-focused, emotion-focused, and active coping were associated with better adjustment (Catz et al., 2002; Pakenham & Rinaldis, 2001) and avoidant coping was related to more psychological distress and lower psychological well-being (Heckman et al., 2004; Smith et al., 2001).

Studies of emotional distress in women with HIV are important because of the potential link with health outcomes. Psychological distress is a barrier to seeking health care in women with HIV (Raveis, Siegel, & Gorey, 1998) and affects adherence to adhere to medication (Boggs, 2002; Catz, Kelly, Bogart, Benotsch, & McAulit, 2000; Mellins et al., 2003). Furthermore, depression has an impact on quality of life and on health (Tate et al., 2003; Tostes et al., 2004). Negative emotional states compromise the immune system and increase susceptibility to disease (Cruess et al., 2003) and there is increasing evidence that psychological distress has a negative impact on the progress of the disease and mortality rates (Farinpour et al., 2003; Kopnisky, Stoff, & Rausch, 2004; Leserman, 2003). Two large prospective studies found that chronically depressed women, in particular had a much higher mortality rate than other women (Cook et al., 2004; Ickovics et al., 2001).

In summary, women with HIV are at high risk for psychological distress. Most studies focused on depressive symptoms; few examined more transient emotional distress such as mood state. Personal characteristics particularly social support, interpersonal conflict, spirituality, and various demographic characteristics have been related to psychological distress. Perception of health, health problems, and time since diagnosis have also been associated with distress, however, few studies included variables assessing the individual's response to having HIV in their models. Therefore, given the impact that psychological distress can have on women with HIV, there is a need to systematically explore multiple factors associated with emotional distress in order to develop interventions to improve psychological well-being and physical health. With the high rate of HIV infection in African American women, there is an urgent need to learn more about emotional distress in this population.

The purpose of this study, then, was to identify factors associated with emotional distress in African American women with HIV. The conceptual model for this study was based on the existing empirical literature and on an adaptation of the Transactional Stress and Coping Model developed by Thompson and colleagues for studies of maternal adjustment to a child's chronic health problem (Thompson & Gustafson, 1996). In our model, the diagnosis of HIV is viewed as a chronic stressor in the lives of the women that leads to emotional distress including both transient mood states and depressive symptoms. These stress responses are influenced by personal characteristics (demographic factors, social conflict, social support, and spirituality), health-related factors (perception of health, physical health and mental health problems, and years since diagnosis), and cognitive/coping responses to having HIV (stigma, worry, and emotion focused coping strategies).

METHODS

Participants and Setting

Participants were 109 African American women who were enrolled in a clinical intervention study, the HIV Self-Care Management Intervention, designed to help mothers of young children with HIV learn how to assess, prevent, and manage HIV-related health problems (Miles et al., 2003). Recruitment occurred in one of two adult infectious disease clinics based in a university tertiary care health center and in community agencies. Women had to be the primary caregiver of a child under the age of 9, be diagnosed with HIV but not have AIDS defining illness, and be African American. Ninety-two mothers and 17 grandmothers were included.

The mean age of the women was 36 with a range from 18 to 66 (see Table 1). About a third (39%) were married or living with a partner. Most (64%) were high school graduates (range 7 to 18 years) and most (68%) did not work. Income of the participants was low; only 8% had incomes over $15,000 and most were receiving public assistance including

TABLE 1. Descriptive Statistics for Predictor and Outcome Variables

Variable	N	Mean (sd) or count (%)	Range
PERSONAL CHARACTERISTICS			
Age (years)	109	36.0 (8.6)	18.3, 65.5
Married or Partnered	108	42 (38.9%)	No,yes
High School Graduate	109	70 (64.2%)	No,yes
Income > $15,000	86	7 (8.1%)	No,yes
Employed	108	33 (30.6%)	No,yes
Public Housing	102	21 (20.6%)	No,yes
Rural (town < 25,000)	107	47 (43.9%)	Urban,rural
Number of children living with	109	2.20 (1.43)	0, 7
Social support	106	3.90 (0.91)	1.6, 5.0
Social conflict	109	2.66 (0.84)	1, 4.8
Spirituality	108	5.56 (0.77)	1.8, 6.0
HEALTH-RELATED FACTORS			
Perception of Health	107	3.19 (1.05)	1, 5
Number of other health problems	109	0.13 (0.10)	0, 36
Years since diagnosis	108	5.3 (2.91)	1,16
Mental health problems	109	0.66 (0.87)	0, 3
RESPONSE TO ILLNESS			
HIV Stigma	109	1.97 (0.68)	1, 3.8
HIV Worry	109	1.95 (1.19)	0, 4
Emotion-Focused Coping	109	3.59 (0.43)	2.18, 4.45
OUTCOME VARIABLES			
Center for Epidemiologic Depression Scale	109	16.80 (10.98)	0,47
Profile of Mood States: Depressed Mood	108	16.44 (14.56)	0,58
Profile of Mood States: Tension	108	11.67 (7.83)	0,32
Profile of Mood States: Anger	108	12.47 (11.17)	0,43
Profile of Mood States: Fatigue	108	9.95 (7.27)	0,28
Profile of Mood States: Confusion	108	8.63 (5.67)	0,24
Profile of Mood States: Vigor	109	17.43 (7.73)	0,32

Medicaid (74%), SSI or social security (64%), and/or food stamps (56%). While the majority of women lived in medium sized cities, about half resided in rural areas and small towns. The women had a mean of 2.2 children living with them (range 1 to 7).

The women had been diagnosed with HIV from 1 to 14 years (M = 5.3 years). Most learned of their HIV diagnosis through routine HIV testing or while pregnant; a few were tested because they were ill. Most women (87%) said they acquired HIV through heterosexual contact with an infected partner. Few (6%) reported IV drug use as the source of transmission. Some were unaware of how they got HIV.

Data Collection Methods

Data were collected via self-report questionnaires at time of enrollment into the study, prior to randomization into the intervention. Data collection methods assessed emotional distress, personal characteristics, health-related characteristics, and cognitive/coping responses.

Emotional Distress. Emotional distress, in this study, included depressive symptoms and mood state. The Center for Epidemiologic Studies Depression Scale (CESD) was used to assess depressive symptoms (Radloff, 1977). This 20-item scale assesses the frequency of the occurrence of feelings or behaviors such as the blues, not feeling as good as others or thinking one's life was a failure. Items are rated on a 4-point scale ranging from 0 (rarely) to 3 (frequently). The CESD is computed as the sum of individual items; the range is 0 to 60. Higher scores indicate more symptoms and a score of 16 indicates risk for depression (Radloff, 1977). The CESD is widely used in studies of individuals with HIV. However, Kalichman, Rompa and Cage (2000) suggest that CESD scores might be affected by HIV-related symptoms, while Belkin and colleagues (Belkin, Fleishman, Stein, Piette, & Mor, 1992) view concern about the effect of physical symptoms on depression exaggerated. We examined the psychometric properties of the CESD with and without physical symptom items and found no differences (Miles et al., 1997). Therefore, we used all items in analysis. In a study of 87 low-income African American mothers with HIV, Cronbach's alpha was .90 (Miles et al., 1997). In this study, Cronbach's alpha was .88.

The Profile of Mood States (POMS) measures transient mood states (McNair, Lorr, & Droppleman, 1971). Six mood states are rated: depressed mood (9 items), tension (15 items), anger (12 items), fatigue (7 items), confusion (7 items) and vigor (8 items). Participants rate each mood state using a 5-point Likert scale ranging from 0 (not at all) to 4 (extremely). Summated scores for each mood state as well as an overall mood score are computed. The range of scores for each mood state varies according to the number of items. Higher scores indicate a more negative mood except for vigor where higher scores indicate more vigor. The POMS has been used extensively with adults with cancer and other chronic illness including HIV (Nyenhius, Yamamoto, Luchetta, Terrien, & Parmentier, 1999). The internal consistency reliabilities in our sample are as follows: .94 for depressed mood, .84 for tension, .91 for anger, .89 for fatigue, .78 for confusion, and .84 for vigor.

Personal Characteristics. Personal and family demographic variables collected included age, partnership status, educational level, income level, employment status, public housing, number of children, and location of residence (rural or urban). Additional personal variables included social support, social conflict, and spirituality. The Medical Outcomes Study-Social Support Survey (MOS-SSS) (Sherbourne & Stewart, 1991) included items assessing emotional, informational, and tangible support, positive social interaction, and affection. Subjects rate the availability of someone in their network for support in these domains using a 5-point rating scale ranging from 1 (none of the time) to 5 (all of the time). Higher scores indicate more support. Cronbach's alpha in our study was .96.

The Social Conflicts Scale (Girdler, Pederson, Stern, & Light, 1993) assessed conflict associated with interpersonal relationships. Participants rate the frequency of selected negative relationships with family or friends using a 5-point scale ranging from 1 (no, never) to 5 (yes, all the time). Higher scores indicate more conflict. Cronbach's alpha in our sample was .70.

The *Religious Well-Being* was used to assess spirituality (Ellison, 1983). Only the spiritual well-being subscale that measures relatedness to God in personal terms was used. Subjects indicate their agreement with 10 statements using a 6-point Likert scale. Higher mean scores indicate a higher level of spirituality. Cronbach's alpha in our sample was .95.

Health-Related Variables. Health variables included perception of health, physical and mental health problems and years since diagnosis. Perception of health was measured using the perception of health subscale of the Medical Outcomes Survey–HIV scale (MOS-HIV) (Wu et al., 1991). Participants use a 5-point rating scale to indicate the degree to which 5 statements related to health are true for them; 2 items are in reverse directions and are recoded for analysis so that higher mean scores indicate a better perception of health. Cronbach's alpha in our study was .80.

Physical health and mental health problems were assessed using a Health Questionnaire developed for the study. Participants checked off whether or not they had any of a list of 22 health problems. This number was converted to a proportion of the total 22 health problems for analysis. To assess mental health, participants rated whether they had problems with nerves, alcohol, and/or drugs in the past 12 months. The number of mental health problems reported ranged from 0 to 3.

Response to Illness. The cognitive and coping response of women to their HIV diagnosis was assessed by measuring perceptions of stigma, worry about HIV, and emotion-focused coping strategies. Stigma was measured using the Demi HIV Stigma Scale (Demi, Bakeman, Sowell, & Moneyham, 2001). Subjects indicate how often they have perceived 12 statements on the tool using a rating scale from 1 (not at all) to 4 (often). Higher mean scores indicate more perceived stigma. Cronbach's alpha in a sample of 264 HIV-positive women was .81 (Demi et al., 2001). In a study of African American mothers with HIV, Cronbach's alpha scores ranged from .77 to .84 and stigma was a significant predictor of depression (Miles et al., 1997). Cronbach's alpha in this study was .87.

Worry about HIV was assessed using the HIV Worry Scale (Miles et al., 2003). The 9 items on the scale assess worry about various aspects of having HIV including current and future health status and dying; items were identified from interviews with women who had HIV. Participants rate each item on a scale ranging from 0 (not at all) to 4 (very much) with higher mean scores indicating greater worry. Cronbach's alpha for this study was .91.

Emotion-focused coping, defined as strategies used to reduce emotional distress, was measured using a scale developed for this study based on the coping literature (Miles et al., 2003). Participants rated the frequency with which they used 5 strategies using a 4-point rating scale ranging from 1 (always) to 4 (never). Mean scores were computed with higher scores indicating more use of strategies. Cronbach's alpha was .83 in this study.

Procedures

This study was approved by the institutional review boards at each of the university medical centers and through a single program assurance for community groups. Mothers were recruited during a clinic visit with the assistance of staff, or via contact with community leaders. The research assistants told the woman about purpose of the study and what was involved. If the mother agreed to be in the study, she signed an IRB approved consent form.

RESULTS

The amount of missing information (less than 75% of data on any given scale) was low. To adjust missing responses in a scale, summed scales were computed as the number of items multiplied by the mean score of non-missing items.

The CESD scores ranged from 0 to 47 with a mean score of 16.8. Thus, the mean scores for the CESD are just above the cut-off indicating risk for depression. All of the POMS scores indicated higher distress than the adult norms for the scale; depressive mood and anger were higher than scores of adult women with cancer. The pairwise correlations among the POMS variables were moderate to high (range .39 to .82) with the exception of correlations involving POMS-vigor (range −.03 to −.32). This supports the use of a multivariate modeling approach for analysis of the POMS scores. Table 1 shows the means, standard deviations, and ranges of predictor and outcome variables.

Pearson correlations between personal characteristics, health-related variables, and cognitive coping variables and the emotional distress outcome variables revealed that education, income, employment status, urban or rural residence, and number of children were not statistically significantly (unadjusted correlation p. > .05) correlated with CESD scores and were eliminated from the CESD analysis. Likewise, these same variables with the exception of employment status were not significantly correlated at least one of the six mood state scores and were eliminated from the POMS analysis.

Factors Associated with Depression

A linear regression model for CESD was determined by applying a stepwise selection process to the predictor variables that were significantly correlated with CESD. A selection to enter criterion of p = .25 and a selection to stay criterion of p = .05 were used. This stepwise process was separately applied to three groupings of predictor variables: personal characteristics (age, public housing, social support social conflicts, spirituality), health-related variables (general health perception, physical health problems, mental health problems, years since diagnosis), and cognitive/coping responses (stigma, worry, emotion-focused coping).

The resulting predictors from each of these two procedures were then combined, and a final model was determined through a third stepwise selection process.

Six independent variables, including the intercept, were selected into this final model. Their estimates, standard errors and p values are given in Table 2. Only emotion-focused coping was not significant in the final model. The final model explained 53% of the variation in CESD (R^2 = .53). Findings revealed that younger age, more social conflict and less social support, lower perception of health, and more HIV worry are associated with higher depressive symptoms.

Factors Associated with Mood State

For the POMs variables, since the six outcome variables are from the same scale we employed a three-step process to identify a common set of predictors while still providing unique estimates for each model. As noted earlier, variables that were not significantly related to any of the POMs outcomes were omitted. Next, stepwise selection procedures were implemented for multiple linear regression models on each outcome separately with a selection to enter criterion of $p = .25$ and a selection to stay criterion of $p = .05$. Those covariates absent from all six resulting models were omitted from further consideration. In the third and final step, the remaining variables were entered into multivariate linear regression models (assuming an unstructured covariance matrix) to provide simultaneous fits of the six multiple linear regression models. A backwards elimination model was used to reduce the number of statistical tests; the criterion for covariates to stay in the model was .05. This process was repeated sepa-

TABLE 2. Linear Regression Model for Center for Epidemiologic Studies Depression Scale: Parameter Estimates, Standard Errors and p-values

Variable	Estimates	s.e.	P-value
Intercept	28.60	7.08	< .001
Age	−0.28	0.10	.006
Social conflicts	4.11	1.10	< .001
Social support	−2.73	0.96	.005
Perception of health	−2.19	0.84	.010
HIV Worry	2.40	0.83	.005

R squared = 0.53

rately for personal characteristics, health-related variables, and cognitive/coping responses. The predictors that were significant from these three models were combined to provide the predictor variables for the final model. Each covariate was evaluated using a six degrees of freedom test for the null hypothesis that the covariate's 6 beta coefficients, one for each POMS subscale, are simultaneously equal to zero. This gives equal emphasis to each of the six POMS outcomes as being indicators of emotional distress in the women.

Applying stepwise regression procedures to each POMS subscale, a total of 7 variables were identified for further consideration. These included 5 personal characteristics (employed, public housing, social support, social conflicts, spirituality), one health-related variable (perception of health) and one cognitive/coping response (HIV worry).

The results of the final step of the model selection procedure are given in Table 3. Of the variables included as predictors in step 2, only spirituality failed to stay in the multivariate model. However, as shown in Table 3 the strength of these associations varied across POMS subscales. Living in public housing and higher social conflicts and HIV worry were significantly associated with depressed mood. Higher social conflicts and HIV worry and being unemployed were associated with more tension. Living in public housing, higher social conflicts and HIV worry were associated with higher anger scores. Public housing, a lower perception of health, and more HIV worry were associated with higher fatigue scores. Public housing and higher HIV worry were associated with higher conflict scores and higher social support was related to higher vigor scores. The percent of variation explained ranged from 36% to 50% across five of the POMS subscales, but only 25% of the variation was explained for the vigor scale.

DISCUSSION

Findings indicate that personal factors have a significant impact on both depressive symptoms and mood state. Younger age, more social conflict, and less social support were associated with higher depressive symptom scores. Regarding mood state, more social conflict was related to depressed mood, tension, and anger; more social support was associated with vigor; public housing was associated with depressed mood, anger, fatigue, and confusion; and unemployment was associated with tension. Findings differ from many studies that found social support more strongly associated with mental health and emotional distress (Catz et al.,

TABLE 3. Linear Regression Model for the Profile of Mood States Scales: Parameter Estimates, Standard Errors and p-values

Variable	POMS Depressed mood	POMS Tension	POMS Anger	POMS Fatigue	POMS Confusion	POMS Vigor	Overall[a]
Intercept	4.86	2.52	−8.66	9.08	10.02**	.53	< .001
	(8.07)	(4.12)	(6.53)	(3.72)	(3.19)	(4.87)	
Employed	−3.12	−3.87**	−3.33	−.99	−1.79	2.43	.036
	(2.46)	(1.26)	(1.99)	(1.14)	(.97)	(1.49)	
Public Housing	7.25*	2.76	6.96**	5.52**	2.38*	1.64	.004
	(2.83)	(1.45)	(2.29)	(1.31)	(1.11)	(1.72)	
Social Support	−1.53	.07	.48	−.19	−.85	2.99**	.004
	(1.30)	(.66)	(1.05)	(.60)	(.51)	(.79)	
Social Conflicts	4.56**	2.68**	4.80**	1.23	.42	.98	.001
	(1.52)	(.78)	(1.23)	(.70)	(.60)	(.92)	
Perception of Health	−1.06	−.70	.59	−1.88**	−.87	1.13	< .001
	(1.18)	(.60)	(.96)	(.54)	(.47)	(.71)	
HIV Worry	4.21**	2.45**	2.14*	1.79**	1.92**	−.95	< .001
	(1.11)	(.57)	(.90)	(.51)	(.43)	(.67)	
R-squared	.44	.50	.36	.49	.43	.25	

*p-value < .05, **p-value < .01.
[a]Overall column gives the p-value for the test that the 6 regression coefficients in that row are simultaneously equal to 0.

2002; Fleishman et al., 2000; Gielen et al., 2001; Hudson et al., 2001; Lapedagne et al., 2000; Mellins et al., 2003; Pakenham & Rinaldis, 2001; Serovich et al., 2001; Silver et al., 2003) in that it was only related to one variable (vigor). It may be that social conflict is a more salient variable to measure in low-income women; it was related to depressive symptoms, depressed mood, tension, and anger. This complements other findings about unsupportive relationships as a factor associated with depression (Fleishman et al., 2000; Schrimshaw, 2003). Two variables associated with poverty, unemployment and public housing, related to various mood states but not to depressive symptoms. This suggests that the two constructs are different; depressive symptoms may reflect more prolonged distress while mood state reflects more immediate distress. The finding that spirituality was not related to emotional distress is likely related to a lack of variability in this measure; most women rated their spirituality high. In addition, the instrument likely was not culturally sensitive for African American women.

It is interesting to note that only one health variable was related to emotional distress, namely perception of health, significantly related to both depressive symptoms and fatigue. This supports the importance of measuring perception of health as well as other more objective data about health. That other health problems were not salient may be related to the relatively young age of the women. That years since diagnosis was not significant mirrors other findings (Ciesla & Roberts, 2001). A major limitation of the study was that HIV-related symptoms were not measured. The tool used in this study to measure symptom distress had poor reliabilities and could not be used in analysis. Furthermore, attempts to measure CD4 counts and HIV-1 RNA were not successful due to the difficulty getting access to records and the irregular patterns of when these tests were done. Further research is needed to identify reliable self-report measures of HIV-related health problems and symptoms and to relate these to emotional distress.

The only response variable that was significant was worry about HIV; it was significantly related to all of the emotional distress variables except vigor. Worry and stigma were both highly correlated with the outcome measures and with each other so worry may have taken up the variance related to stigma. While emotional focused coping was not significant in the final models, it was also significantly correlated with all of the outcome measures providing some support that emotion-focused coping is associated with less emotional distress.

This paper supports other authors who have recently identified the urgent need to provide mental health services to women with HIV. However, rather than assessing and referring women who are highly distressed to mental health clinics, such services need to become an integral part of HIV care in order to prevent serious mental health problems and to help women adapt to and learn to live with their diagnosis. Research is needed to develop and assess the impact of services that are effective in increasing health related self-care and health care seeking behaviors and adherence to medications. Such approaches should ultimately decrease complications and increase survival of women with HIV.

REFERENCES

Belkin, G.S., Fleishman, J.A., Stein, M.D., Piette, J., & Mor, V. (1992). Physical symptoms and depressive symptoms among individuals with HIV infection. *Psychosomatics, 33*, 416-427.

Bennetts, A., Shaffer, N., Manopaiboon, C., Chaiyakul, P., Siriwasin, W., Mock, P. et al. (1999). Determinants of depression and HIV-related worry among HIV-positive women who have recently given birth, Bangkok, Thailand. *Social Science & Medicine, 49,* 737-749.

Bing, E.G., Burnam, M.A., Longshore, D., Fleishman, J.A., Sherbourne, C.D., London, A.S. et al. (2001). Psychiatric disorders and drug use among human immunodeficiency virus-infected adults in the United States. *Archives of General Psychiatry, 58,* 721-728.

Blalock, A.C., McDaniel, J.S., & Farber, E.W. (2002). Effect of employment on quality of life and psychological functioning in patients with HIV/AIDS. *Psychosomatics, 43,* 400-404.

Boggs, W. (2002). Depression impairs adherence to HAART regimen by HIV-infected women. *Journal of Acquired Immune Deficiency Syndrome, 30,* 401-409.

Catz, S.L., Gore-Felton, C., & McClure, J.B. (2002). Psychological distress among minority and low-income women living with HIV. *Behavioral Medicine, 28,* 53-60.

Catz, S.L., Kelly, J.A., Bogart, L.M., Benotsch, E.G., & McAulit, T.L. (2000). Patterns, correlates, and barriers to medication adherence among persons prescribed new treatments for HIV disease. *Health Psychology, 19,* 124-133.

Ciesla, J.A., & Roberts, J.E. (2001). Meta-analysis of the relationship between HIV infection and risk for depressive disorders. *American Journal of Psychiatry, 158,* 725-730.

Coleman, C.L., & Holzemer, W.L. (1999). Spirituality, psychological well-being, and HIV symptoms for African Americans living with HIV. *Journal of Community Psychology, 22,* 224-230.

Cook, J.A., Grey, D., Burke, J., Cohen, M.H., Gurtman, A.C., Richardson, J.L. et al. (2004). Depressive symptoms and AIDS-related mortality among a multisite cohort of HIV-positive women. *American Journal of Public Health, 94,* 1133-1140.

Cruess, D.G., Douglas, S.D., Petitto, J.M., Leserman, J., Ten Have, T., Gettes, D. et al. (2003). Association of depression, CD8+ T lymphocytes and natural killer cell activity: Implications for morbidity and mortality in human immunodeficiency virus disease. *Current Psychiatry Reports, 5,* 445-450.

Demi, A.S., Bakeman, R., Sowell, R., & Moneyham, L. (2001). *Psychometric evaluation of the Demi HIV Stigma Scale.* Unpublished manuscript submitted for publication.

Ellison, C. (1983). Spiritual well-being: Conceptualization and measurement. *Journal of Psychology and Theology, 11,* 330-340.

Farinpour, R., Miller, E.N., Satz, P., Selnes, O.A., Cohen, B.A., Becker, J.T. et al. (2003). Psychosocial risk factors of HIV morbidity and mortality: Findings from the Multicenter AIDS Cohort Study (MACS). *Journal of Clinical Experimental Neuropsychology, 25,* 654-670.

Fleishman, J.A., Sherbourne, C.D., Crysal, S., Collins, R.L., Marshall, G.N., Kelly, M. et al. (2000). Coping, conflictual social interactions, social support, and mood among HIV-infected persons. *American Journal of Community Psychology, 28,* 421-453.

Franke, G.H., Jager, H., Stacker, K.H., & Beyer, B. (1995). Between isolation and new hope: The psychosocial status of HIV-infected women. *Psychotherapy, Psychosomatic Medicine, & Psychology, 45,* 310-320.

Gielen, A.C., McDonnell, K.A., Wu, A.W., O'Campo, P., & Faden, R. (2001). Quality of life among women living with HIV: The importance of violence, social support, and self-care behaviors. *Social Science and Medicine, 52,* 315-322.

Girdler, S.S., Pederson, C.A., Stern, R.A., & Light, K.C. (1993). Menstrual cycle and premenstrual syndrome: Modifiers of cardiovascular reactivity in women. *Health Psychology, 12,* 180-192.

Heckman, T.G., Anderson, E.S., Sikkema, K.J., Kochman, A., Kalichman, S.C., & Anderson, T. (2004). Emotional distress in nonmetropolitan persons living with HIV disease enrolled in a telephone-delivered, coping improvement group intervention. *Health Psychology, 23,* 94-100.

Hudson, A.L., Lee, K.A., Miramontes, H., & Portillo, C.J. (2001). Social interactions, perceived support, and level of distress in HIV-positive women. *Journal of the Association of Nurses in AIDS Care, 12,* 68-76.

Ickovics, J.R., Hamburger, M.E., Vlahov, D., Schoenbaum, E.E., Schuman, P., Boland, R.J. et al. (2001). Mortality, CD4 cell count decline, and depressive symptoms among HIV-seropositive women: Longitudinal analysis from the HIV Epidemiologic Research Study. *Journal of the American Medical Association, 285,* 1466-1474.

Kalichman, S.C., Rompa, D., & Cage, M. (2000). Distinguishing between overlapping somatic symptoms of depression and HIV disease in people living with HIV-AIDS. *Journal of Nervous and Mental Disease, 188,* 662-670.

Kaplan, M.S., Marks, G., & Mertens, S.B. (1997). Distress and coping among women with HIV infection: Preliminary findings from a multiethnic sample. *American Journal of Orthopsychiatry, 67,* 80-91.

Kopnisky, K.L., Stoff, D.M., & Rausch, D.M. (2004). Workshop report: The effect of psychological variables on the progress of HIV-1 disease. *Brain, Behavior, and Immunity, 18,* 246-261.

Lapedagne, T., Ferriere, J.P., Lacoste, D., & Verdoux, H. (2000). Anxiety and depression among HIV-positive subjects: Prevalence and risk factors. *Annals Medico-Psychologiques, 158,* 21-32.

Leserman, J. (2003). HIV disease progression: Depression, stress, and possible mechanisms. *Biological Psychiatry, 54,* 295-306.

McClure, J.B., Catz, S.L., Prejean, J., Branteley, P.J., & Jones, G.N. (1996). Factors associated with depression in a heterogeneous HIV-infected sample. *Journal of Psychosomatic Research, 40,* 407-415.

McNair, D. M., Lorr, M., & Droppleman, L. F. (1971). *Manual for the Profile of Mood States.* San Diego: Educational and Industrial Testing Service.

Mellins, C.A., Kang, E., Leu, C.S., Havens, J.F., & Chesney, M.A. (2003). Longitudinal study of mental health and psychosocial predictors of medical treatment adherence in mothers living with HIV disease. *AIDS Patient Care, 17,* 407-416.

Miles, M.S., Holditch-Davis, D., Burchinal, P., Wasilewski, Y., & Christian, B. (1996). Personal, family, and health-related correlates of depressive symptoms in mothers with HIV. *Journal of Family Psychology, 11,* 23-34

Miles, M.S., Holditch-Davis, D., Eron, J., Black, B.P., Pedersen, C., & Harris, D. (2003). An HIV self-care symptom management intervention for African American mothers. *Nursing Research, 52,* 350-360.

Moneyham, L., Sowell, R., Seals, B., & Demi, A. (2000). Depressive symptoms among African American women with HIV disease. *Scholarly Inquiry for Nursing Practice, 14*, 9-39.

Morrison, M.F., Pettito, J.M., Ten Have, T., Gettes, D.R., Chiappini, M.S., Weber, A.L. et al. (2002). Depressive and anxiety disorders in women with HIV infection. *American Journal of Psychiatry, 159*, 789-796.

Nyenhuis, D.L., Yamamoto, C., Luchetta, T., Terrien, A., & Parmentier, A. (1999). Adult and geriatric normative data and validation of the Profile of Mood States. *Journal of Clinical Psychology, 55*, 79-86.

Orlando, M., Burnam, M.A., Beckman, R., Morton, S.C., London, A.S., Bing, E.G. et al. (2002). Re-estimating the prevalence of psychiatric disorders in a nationally representative sample of persons receiving care for HIV: Results from the HIV Cost and Services Utilization Study. *International Journal of Methods of Psychiatric Research, 11*, 75-82.

Pakenham, K.I., & Rinaldis, M. (2001). The role of illness, resources, appraisal, and coping strategies in adjustment to HIV/AIDS: The direct and buffering effects. *Journal of Behavioral Medicine, 24*, 259-279.

Radloff, L. (1977). The CES-D scale: A self report depression scale for research in the general population. *Applied Psychological Measurement, 1*, 385-401.

Raveis, V.H., Siegel, K., & Gorey, E. (1998). Factors associated with HIV-infected women's delay in seeking medical care. *AIDS Care, 10*, 549-562.

Schrimshaw, E.W. (2003). Relationship-specific unsupportive social interactions and depressive symptoms among women living with HIV/AIDS: Direct and moderating effects. *Journal of Behavioral Medicine, 26*, 297-313.

Serovich, J.M., Kimerly, J.A., Mosack, K.E., & Lewis, T.L. (2001). The role of family and friend social support in reducing emotional distress among HIV-positive women. *AIDS Care, 13*, 335-341.

Sherbourne, C.D,, & Stewart, A.L. (1991). The MOS Social Support Survey. *Social Science and Medicine, 32*, 705-714.

Silver, E.J., Bauman, L.J., Camacho, S., & Hudis, J. (2003). Factors associated with psychological distress in urban mothers with late-state HIV/AIDS. *AIDS Behavior, 7*, 421-431.

Smith, L., Feaster, D.J., Prado, G., Kamin, M., Blaney, N., & Szapocznik, J. (2001). The psychological functioning of HIV + and HIV- African American recent mothers. *AIDS and Behavior, 5*, 219-231

Tate, D. et al. (2003). The impact of apathy and depression on quality of life in patients infected with HIV. *AIDS Patient Care, 17*, 115-120.

Thompson, R.J., & Gustafson, K.E. (1996). *Adaptation to chronic childhood illness.* WDC: American Psychological Association.

Tostes, M.A., Chalub, M., & Botega, N.J. (2004). The quality of life of HIV-infected women is associated with psychiatric morbidity. *AIDS Care, 16*, 177-186.

Wu, A. W., Rubin, H. R., Mathews, W. C., Ware, J. E., Brysk, L. T., Hardy, W. D., Bozzette, S. A., Spector, S. A., & Richman, D. D. (1991). A health status questionnaire using 30 items from the Medical Outcomes Survey. *Medical Care, 29*, 786-798.

doi:10.1300/J005v33n01_04

Unsafe Sex:
Do Feelings Matter?

Celia M. Lescano
Larry K. Brown

Brown University Medical School
Rhode Island Hospital

Paul M. Miller

Psychological Care Associates

Kristie L. Puster

Carolina Mountain Psychiatry

SUMMARY. The purpose of this study was to investigate the relationships among self-efficacy for condom use during distress (SE-Condom Distress), self-efficacy related to general HIV prevention skills (SE-HIV), and HIV risk behaviors, attitudes, and knowledge. Two hundred and twenty two adolescents with psychiatric disorders between 13 and 18 years-old participated. Participants completed measures related to HIV Self-Efficacy, HIV Attitudes, and Sexual Behaviors. Self-efficacy for condom use during distress (SE-Condom Distress) was significantly associated with more HIV protective behaviors. Controlling for ob-

Address correspondence to: Celia M. Lescano, Brown University School of Medicine, Bradley/Hasbro Research Center,1 Hoppin Street, Coro West, Suite 240, Providence, RI 02903 (E-mail: clescano@lifespan.org).

Research was supported by NIMH grant R01 MH61149.

[Haworth co-indexing entry note]: "Unsafe Sex: Do Feelings Matter?" Lescano, Celia M. et al. Co-published simultaneously in *Journal of Prevention & Intervention in the Community* (The Haworth Press, Inc.) Vol. 33, No.1/2, 2007, pp. 51-62; and: *HIV: Issues with Mental Health and Illness* (ed: Michael B. Blank, and Marlene M. Eisenberg) The Haworth Press, Inc., 2007, pp. 51-62. Single or multiple copies of this article are available for a fee from The Haworth Document Delivery Service [1-800-HAWORTH, 9:00 a.m. - 5:00 p.m. (EST). E-mail address: docdelivery@haworthpress.com].

served covariates, SE-Condom Distress was the only variable significantly associated with consistent condom use in a multiple logistic
regression (OR = 2.43). Self-efficacy regarding condom use during affective arousal is closely associated with HIV-related attitudes and behaviors. Clinicians need to be alert to subtle signs of distress as adolescents
contemplate safer sexual behavior. doi:10.1300/J005v33n01_05   *[Article
copies available for a fee from The Haworth Document Delivery Service:
1-800-HAWORTH.   E-mail   address: <docdelivery@haworthpress.com>
Website: <http://www.HaworthPress.com> © 2007 by The Haworth Press, Inc.
All rights reserved.]*

KEYWORDS. Adolescents, HIV, safe sex behaviors, distress

Adolescents and young adults currently account for 50% of new HIV
infections on an annual basis (CDC, 2001). Unsafe sexual behavior that
places adolescents at risk for HIV is related to factors such as emotionality
(e.g., distress and affect dysregulation), cognitions (e.g., low self-efficacy), family influences, and peer norms (Brooks, Harris, Thrall, &
Woods, 2002; Brown, DiClemente, & Reynolds, 1991; DiClemente et
al., 2001). This paper focuses on two of these important influences; affect
regulation and low self-efficacy. As described below, although the importance of self-efficacy in influencing sexual behavior is widely ac-
knowledged, much less is understood of the association between distress
and HIV risk.

Successful regulation of affect can be defined as responding with a
range of emotions in a way that allows one to react spontaneously as well
as to suppress immediate reactions when necessary. In Sheeber, Allen,
Davis, and Sorensen's (2000) micro-analysis of interactions between adolescents and their mothers, adolescents who had more difficulty shifting
out of a depressive state were more likely to have an ongoing affective disorder than those with less difficulty. In most studies, affect dysregulation
is inferred by the presence of psychological symptoms. For example, depression and dysphoria predicted substance abuse in a sample of homeless adolescents (MacLean, Paradise, & Cauce, 1999), suicide attempts
among a nonclinical sample of adolescents (Fritsch, Donaldson, Spirito,
& Plummer, 2000) and physical violence and use of tobacco (Brooks et
al., 2002).

Distress may also lead to HIV risk behaviors (e.g., sharing of self-cut-
ting instruments, unprotected intercourse), though the evidence for an association between distress and HIV-specific risk is limited (Crepaz &

Marks, 2001; Kalichman & Weinhardt, 2001). Recent research supporting this relationship comes from a community sample of adolescents (DiClemente et al., 2001). In this study, adolescents with significant psychological distress assessed at baseline were significantly more likely six months later to have had unprotected vaginal sex, to have had non-monogamous male sex partners, to have not used any form of contraception, and were more likely to have become pregnant. In addition to general psychological distress, psychological distress during sexual situations may precipitate risk behavior. Adolescents with difficulties with affect dysregulation may become overwhelmed with distress in sexual situations because of relationship concerns (e.g., fear of rejection), previous traumatic sexual experiences, or low self-esteem (e.g., because of little motivation to keep oneself healthy) (Brown et al., 1997).

Another key construct in predicting health-promoting behaviors is self-efficacy, the perception that one can engage in protective behaviors (Bandura, 1986; Bandura, 1994). A range of protective behaviors is necessary in order to protect oneself from HIV, including buying condoms, carrying condoms, discussing condom use and safer sex with your partner, and using condoms correctly. While not all of these aspects of HIV prevention have been studied specifically, condom self-efficacy, defined as the belief in one's ability to effectively use condoms, has been found to be an important predictor of engaging in protective behaviors in several studies (Basen-Engquist & Parcel, 1992; Brown, Danovsky, Lourie, DiClemente, & Ponton, 1997). For example, Basen-Engquist and Parcel (1992) found that condom self-efficacy predicted condom use frequency after controlling for attitudes and perceptions of peer norms towards safer sex and sexual abstinence. In another study, Kasen, Vaughan, and Walter (1992) found that among a sample of tenth graders, those students with higher condom self-efficacy were five times more likely to report using condoms consistently than their less confident peers.

Our ongoing work suggests that condom self-efficacy may be an important domain to consider in designing HIV prevention interventions for adolescents. This project investigates HIV prevention among adolescents with psychiatric disorders, a group at high risk because of the prevalence of various risk behaviors (Baker & Mossman, 1991; DiClemente & Ponton, 1993; Donenberg, Emerson, Bryant, Wilson, & Weber-Shifrin, 2001). In an intervention study with adolescents in intensive psychiatric treatment, adolescents participated in role-plays that were videotaped and reviewed (Brown, Lourie et al., 2000). These role-plays were designed to give adolescents practice with, and direct feedback on, their skills in asserting safer sexual behavior. Our clinical observations of the teens in these role-plays suggested that many of them had difficulty being assertive when affective arousal was a salient component of the scenarios.

Adolescents with psychiatric disorders are more likely than community adolescents to have decreased self-efficacy and increased distress, thus providing an opportunity to examine these important associations. In this study, we investigate the associations between the two domains of self-efficacy: condom use during distress (SE-Condom Distress) and general HIV prevention skills (SE-HIV) and HIV risk behaviors (e.g., consistency of condom use), HIV attitudes (e.g., intentions to practice safer sex, perceived susceptibly to HIV infection), and HIV knowledge.

METHOD

Subjects

Participants (N = 222) attended psychiatric day schools; 84.2% of the youths eligible for the study (between the ages of 13 and 18, not psychotic, and able to participate in school activities) were enrolled. Participants had a mean age of 14.83 (SD = 1.48) and 60% were male; 83% were Caucasian, 7% African American, 2% Latino, and 8% endorsed other ethnic groups. The diagnostic range of the sample was similar to that found in other therapeutic settings. The most frequent primary diagnoses were 41% depressive disorders, 30% impulse-control disorders, and 8% PTSD. Forty-one percent of subjects reported a history of sexual abuse.

Procedures

This study was approved by the hospital Institutional Review Board. After describing the study to potential participants, written informed consent was obtained from a parent or guardian, and assent was obtained from the participant. Data were collected at the therapeutic schools using paper-and-pencil measures. Participants were reimbursed with $5 gift certificates for their time and effort.

Measures

All participants completed the following measures at baseline as part of a 12-week intervention to decrease HIV-risk behaviors.

HIV-Related Self-Efficacy. Self-Efficacy for Condom Use During Distress (SE-Condom Distress): This four-item subscale reflected condom self-efficacy ("I am confident I could use a condom when . . . ") during emotional distress such as "I am upset," "I am feeling bad about myself," "I am depressed," and "I am feeling angry." It was derived from a longer scale of condom self-efficacy attitudes and has been used in previous HIV prevention projects to assess self-confidence in condom use and as a measure of change (Brown et al., 2000; Brown, Lourie, Zlotnick, & Cohn, 2000; Prochaska, Redding, Harlow, Rossi, & Velicer, 1994). These four items were selected because of their face validity for distress. In addition, an exploratory principal components factor analysis found that the 4 items loaded on a single factor, with an eigenvalue greater than 1, each with a loading of .75 to .80. It had a final coefficient alpha of 0.92.

HIV Prevention Skills Self-Efficacy (SE-HIV). This 11-item scale measures self-efficacy for the practical skills of HIV prevention. The measure assesses the extent to which teens could engage in specific HIV preventive behaviors such as buying condoms, carrying condoms, discussing condom use and safer sex with your partner, and refusing sex altogether (Lawrence, Levy, & Rubinson, 1990). It has adequate internal consistency (alpha = 0.86).

Other HIV-Related Measures. AIDS knowledge: The 20-item AIDS Knowledge scale (alpha = 0.79) surveys knowledge of routes of transmission, casual contact misconceptions, general information, and course of illness with regard to HIV and AIDS (Brown, DiClemente, & Beausoleil, 1992; Brown & Fritz, 1988).

Perceived Susceptibility. This five-item scale (alpha = 0.51) reflects personal concern about the presence of AIDS in our society (e.g., "I am very nervous about AIDS," and "I am worried that I might already have AIDS"). In young adolescents, change in this scale was found to be the most significant predictor of safe intentions (Brown, Powers, Barone, & Fritz, 1994).

HIV Safe Intentions. This four-item scale reflects an individual's intent to engage in activity that will prevent or avoid HIV infection. These items include: (1) "I'm afraid of getting AIDS, so I will avoid sex." (2) "Even knowing about AIDS, I might shoot drugs with a needle." (3) "If I were to have sex, I would use a condom every time or have my partner use one to protect myself from getting AIDS." (4) "Honestly, if I were sexually active, I probably would have intercourse without protecting myself against AIDS."

General Risk Attitudes. This five-item scale asks questions concerning self-rated impulsivity and sensation-seeking, not specifically pertaining to HIV risk, as a general-risk attitude scale with a Cronbach alpha of 0.68 (Brown, DiClemente, & Park, 1992).

Sexual Behaviors. Sexually active participants (n = 133) reported their behaviors with regard to condoms, in addition to the measures listed above. Sexual activity was defined as engaging in vaginal or anal intercourse lifetime or past 90 days. Adolescents reported whether or not they engaged in consistent condom use ("use condoms all the time"; yes/no), how often they had used condoms in the last six months, if they had used condoms in the last month, and if they had purchased condoms in the last month.

History of Sexual Abuse Checklist. History of sexual abuse was gathered using eight items modeled after Finkelhor's review (Finkelhor, 1979) and has been used in recent projects (Brown, Lourie et al., 2000).

Data Analysis

ANCOVAs to control for age were used to determine the relationship between the self-efficacy scales and attitudes and behaviors. These were followed by multiple logistic regression predicting condom use with both self-efficacy measures and entry of appropriate covariates.

RESULTS

Univariate Analyses

Because of the skewness of the self-efficacy measures, SE-Condom Distress and HIV Prevention Skills Self-Efficacy (SE-HIV), were divided into tertiles to examine the association between self-efficacy and sexual behavior and attitudes. There was no association between scores on either of the two self-efficacy scales and gender, ethnicity, or diagnosis. Older age was associated with increased SE-Condom Distress [15.1 (SD = 1.3) vs. 14.6 (SD = 1.6); t (201) = 2.26, p = .03] and with SE-HIV [15.3 (SD = 1.4) vs. 14.2 (SD = 1.6); t (137) = 4.36, p < .001]. SE-Condom Distress and SE-HIV were unrelated to psychiatric diagnosis or to a history of sexual abuse.

Controlling for age differences with ANCOVAs, tests found that adolescents with higher SE-Condom Distress scores (i.e., higher perceived self-efficacy for condom use during distress) had greater HIV-safe intentions and higher HIV knowledge scores (Table 1). Greater SE-Condom Distress was also significantly associated with the use of condoms over 6 months and a trend towards more consistent condom use (p = .07) and use of condoms in the past month (p = .06).

TABLE 1. Condom Use Self-Efficacy During Distress (SE-Condom Distress) and Risk Behaviors/Attitudes

Measure	Affective Arousal						
	Low Self Efficacy (N = 57)		High Self Efficacy (N = 67)		Analysis		
	Mean	SD	Mean	SD	F	df	p
Scale							
AIDS Knowledge	13.8	2.83	15	2.72	4.53	2	0.005
Perceived Susceptibility	4.09	1.71	4.1	2.15	0.41	2	0.66
HIV Safe Intentions	5.47	1.62	6.1	1.46	15.51	2	0.01
General Risk Attitudes	4.91	2.66	4.13	2.78	1.67	2	0.19
	%	N	%	N	x2	df	p
Item							
Consistent Condom Use	52.6%	20/38	75.0%	39/52	8.63	4	0.071
Use of condoms for 6 months	34.2%	13/38	62.7%	32/51	15.79	4	0.003
Used condoms in past month	17.5%	10/57	32.3%	21/65	3.49	1	0.06
Bought condoms in past month	36.8%	21/57	49.2%	32/65	1.9	1	0.12
History of Sexual Abuse	51.9%	27/52	43.1%	25/58	0.86	1	0.36

Note: N's vary based on sexual activity status, skip patterns, and missing data

A similar pattern was found for SE-HIV. After controlling for age differences with ANCOVAs it was found that those with higher SE-HIV scores had greater AIDS knowledge and less general risk attitudes. Behavioral differences were present but were not as striking as in the previous analysis for SE-Condom Distress. Similar univariate tests (not reported) among just the sexually active adolescents revealed a similar pattern of differences between high and low SE-HIV groups. Among the sexually active, HIV self-efficacy was associated with greater length of time of condom use.

Logistic Regression

A multiple logistic regression for consistent condom use simultaneously examined age, gender, SE-HIV and SE-Condom Distress, using scales split at the median (Model Chi Square (4) = 12.24, n = 133, p = .02). Table 2 indicates that SE-Condom Distress was the only variable significantly associated with consistent condom use (Adjusted OR = 2.4, Wald = 4.17, $p < .05$).

DISCUSSION

This project suggests the importance of self-efficacy during distress in maintaining safer sexual behavior. It is known that affect regulation plays a critical role in other health behaviors but its importance in relation to HIV prevention has not been demonstrated previously. This study found that self-efficacy regarding condom use during affective arousal (SE-Condom Distress) is a specific domain of condom self-efficacy and that it was closely associated with HIV-related attitudes and behaviors. This finding is consistent with the observations of role-plays in which participants were ineffective because of their emotional distress. More importantly, SE-Condom Distress was highly associated with HIV-related attitudes and recent sexual behavior. Given the prime role that self-efficacy has demonstrated in other areas of research, it is not surprising to find this general association. However, the multiple logistic regres-

TABLE 2. Multiple Logistic Regression for Consistent Condom Use (N = 133)

	O. R.	C. I.	P
Variable			
Age			
14 or younger	1		
Older than 14	1.63	.70-3.77	0.26
Gender			
Female	1		
Male	1.66	.73-3.78	0.23
Self-Efficacy: HIV Prevention Skills			
Low	1		
High	1.82	.77-4.29	0.17
Self-Efficacy: Sexual Distress			
Low	1		0.04
High	2.43	1.04 - 5.70	

Note. Scales split at the median
O. R. = Adjusted Odds Ratio
C. I. = Confidence Interval

sion confirms that, controlling for other important variables and general self-efficacy for HIV prevention (SE-HIV), SE-Condom Distress was uniquely related to consistent condom use. These findings suggest that lack of self-efficacy when confronted with the stress of using condoms is a powerful barrier to their use.

The study does not provide data about how to improve self-efficacy during affective arousal. However, there is extensive literature in other areas of health behavior on affect regulation and emotional distress (Lescano, Brown, Puster, & Miller, submitted for review). Simply increasing adolescents' awareness of their distress would not likely be effective because the data are consistent with adolescents being aware of their difficulties with efficacy and this awareness is associated with a lack of condom use. Thus, active strategies to deal with affective management are indicated. Interestingly, SE-Condom Distress was unrelated to a history of sexual abuse or diagnostic categories. This finding suggests that difficulties with affect regulation are widespread and can be found among adolescents with varying histories. It also suggests that skills needed for affect management need not be bound to certain forms of psychopathology but may be viewed best in a general developmental model.

Although this project examined a large number of adolescents with psychiatric disorders, using standard assessment procedure, there are limitations. The sample was a diverse group of adolescents with psychiatric disorders and thus likely to have difficulties with affect management. The extent to which these findings among adolescents with psychiatric disorders are generalizable to a community sample is unknown. However, most high-risk community samples have a significant number of adolescents with psychiatric disorders (Costello, Mustillo, Erkanli, Keeler, & Angold, 2003). Also, distress regarding condom use is a concern of many adolescents, not just those with significant psychiatric issues. It should also be noted that the sample was primarily Caucasian (similar to the population of the state of Rhode Island and those likely to be in psychiatric day schools in Rhode Island), thus limiting the generalizability of these findings for non-Caucasian adolescents. Another potential limitation is the reliance on the self-report of sexual behavior. This study attempted to minimize report bias by the use of multiple indices of sexual risk and assessment procedures done with confidentiality. Also, the general associations between attitudes and behavior were in the expected direction. Finally, it can be noted that the measurement of self-efficacy in the face of distress in sexual situations could have been more complete. As is routine for the measurement of self-efficacy, these items required the adolescent to rate how they would react in a situation rather than how they have reacted. In addition, the level of distress during condom use in any of these situations was not specified, nor were the ways they might have dealt with the distress. Clearly, these data indicate the need for a more detailed examination of the exact situations leading to distress, the extent of distress and the adaptive and maladaptive ways of coping with distress.

There are several implications from this project. Affect regulation in dealing with condom use appears to be an important issue and difficulty with such regulation is likely a barrier towards condom use for many adolescents. Since this factor was unrelated to previous sexual abuse trauma or primary psychiatric diagnosis, it suggests that such difficulties can be encountered in a wide variety of adolescents. Difficulty with distress during condom use is not confined to those that are clinically depressed or emotionally labile. Clinicians and facilitators of interventions need to be alert to subtle signs of distress as adolescents contemplate safer sexual behavior. In fact, the role-plays observed during preliminary work suggested that there were many adolescents with signs of only minimal stress who felt incapable of using condoms. If emotional dysregulation were a problem for an adolescent, this finding would imply the need for interventions to specifically target these skills. Further work is needed to determine how widespread these deficits are and the extent to which they are related to sexual risk behavior in other samples. However, the relationship between distress and other health behaviors suggests that the role of emotions should not be overlooked but should be the focus of further inquiry. Assisting adolescents in managing their emotions may be as important as acquiring practical behavioral skills in order to consistently enact safe sexual behavior.

REFERENCES

Baker, D. & Mossman, D. (1991). Potential HIV exposure in psychiatrically hospitalized adolescent girls. *American Journal of Psychiatry*, 148, 528-530.

Bandura, A. (1986). *Social Foundations of Thought and Action: A Social Cognitive Theory.* Englewood Cliffs, NJ: Prentice-Hall.

Bandura, A. (1994). Social cognitive theory and exercise of control over HIV infection. In R.J. DiClemente (Ed.), *Preventing AIDS: Theories and methods of behavioral interventions. AIDS Prevention and Mental Health* (pp. 25-59). New York, NY: Plenum Press.

Basen-Engquist, K. & Parcel, G. S. (1992). Attitudes, norms, and self-efficacy: A model of adolescents' HIV-related sexual risk behavior. *Health Education Quarterly*, 19, 263-277.

Brooks, T. L., Harris, S. K., Thrall, J. S. & Woods, E. R. (2002). Association of adolescent risk behaviors with mental health symptoms in high school students. *Journal of Adolescent Health*, 31(3), 240-246.

Brown, L., Danovsky, M., Lourie, K., DiClemente, R., & Ponton, L. (1997). Adolescents with psychiatric disorders and the risk of HIV. *Journal of the American Academy of Child and Adolescent Psychiatry*, 36, 1609-1617.

Brown, L., DiClemente, R., & Beausoleil, N. (1992). Comparison of HIV-related knowledge, attitudes, intentions and behaviors among sexually active and abstinent young adolescents. *Journal of Adolescent Health*, 13,140-145.

Brown, L., DiClemente, R., & Park, T. (1992). Predictors of condom use in sexually active adolescents. *Journal of Adolescent Health*, 13, 651-657.

Brown, L., DiClemente, R., & Reynolds, L. (1991). HIV prevention for adolescents: Utility of the Health Belief Model. *AIDS Education and Prevention*, 3, 50-59.

Brown, L., & Fritz, G. (1988). Children's knowledge and attitudes about AIDS. *Journal of the American Academy of Child and Adolescent Psychiatry*, 27, 504-508.

Brown, L. K., Lourie, K. J., & Lescano, C. M. (in preparation). HIV prevention for adolescents with psychiatric disorders: A program evaluation.

Brown, L., Lourie, K., Zlotnick, C., & Cohn, J. (2000). Impact of sexual abuse on the HIV-risk-related behavior of adolescents in intensive psychiatric treatment. *American Journal of Psychiatry*, 157, 1413-1415.

Brown, L., Powers, S., Barone, V., & Fritz, G. (1994). Influences on intentions to abstinence in young adolescents. Annual Meeting of the American Academy of Child and Adolescent Psychiatry, New York, NY.

Brown, L., Schultz, J., Parsons, J., Butler, R., Forsberg, A., Kocik, S., King, G., Manco-Johnson, M., & Aledort, L. (2000). Sexual behavior change among HIV infected adolescents. *Pediatrics*, 106, 22.

Centers for Disease Control (2001). Young People at Risk: HIV/AIDS Among America's Youth.

Costello, E. J., Mustillo, S., Erkanli, A., Keeler, G., & Angold, A. (2003). Prevalence and development of psychiatric disorders in childhood and adolescence. *Archives of General Psychiatry*, 60 (8), 837-844.

Crepaz, N., & Marks, G. (2001). Are negative affective states associated with HIV sexual risk behaviors? A meta-analytic review. *Health Psychology*, 20(4), 291-299.

DiClemente, R. & Ponton, L. (1993). HIV-related risk behaviors among psychiatrically hospitalized adolescents and school-based adolescents. *American Journal of Psychiatry*, 150, 324-325.

DiClemente, R. J., Wingwood, G. M., Crosby, R., Sionean, C., Brown, L., Rothbaum, B., Zimand, E., Cobb, B. K., Harrington, K., & Davies, S. (2001). A prospective study of psychological distress and sexual risk behavior among African American adolescent females. *Pediatrics*, 108(5), 1-6.

Donenberg, G. R., Emerson, E., Bryant, F. B., Wilson, H., & Weber-Shifrin, E. (2001). Understanding AIDS-risk behavior among adolescents in psychiatric care: Links to psychopathology and peer relationships. *Journal of the American Academy of Child and Adolescent Psychiatry*, 40(6), 642-653.

Finkelhor, D. (1979). What's wrong with sex between adults and children? Ethics and the problem of sexual abuse. *American Journal of Orthopsychiatry*, 49(4), 692-697.

Fritsch, S., Donaldson, D., Spirito, A., & Plummer, B. (2000). Personality characteristics of adolescent suicide attempters. *Child Psychiatry and Human Development*, 30, 219-235.

Kalichman, S. C. & Weinhardt, L. (2001). Negative affect and sexual risk behavior: Comment on Crepaz and Marks (2001). *Health Psychology*, 20(4), 300-301.

Kasen, S., Vaughn, R. D., & Walter, H. J. (1992). Self-efficacy for AIDS preventive behaviors among tenth grade students. *Health Education Quarterly, 19*(2), 187-202.

Lawrence, L., Levy, S.R., & Rubinson, L. (1990). Self-efficacy and AIDS prevention for pregnant teens. *Journal of School Health*, 60 (1), 19-24.

Lescano, C., Brown, L., Puster, K., & Miller, P. (submitted for review). Sexual abuse and adolescent HIV risk: A group intervention framework.

MacLean, M.G., Paradise, M. J. & Cauce, A. M. (2000). Substance use and psychological adjustment in homeless adolescents: A test of three models. *American Journal of Community Psychology*, 27, 405-427.

Prochaska, J. & DiClemente, C. (1992). Stages of change in the modification of problem behaviors. In M. Hersen, R. Eisler, & P. Miller (Eds.), *Progress in Behavior Modification* (pp. 183-218). Newbury Park, CA: Sage.

Prochaska, J., Redding, C., Harlow, L., Rossi, J., & Velicer, W. F. (1994). The transtheoretical model of change and HIV prevention: A review. *Health Education Quarterly*, 21, 471-486.

Sheeber, L., Allen, N., Davis, B., & Sorenson, E. (2000). Regulation of negative affect during mother-child problem-solving interactions: Adolescent depressive status and family processes. *Journal of Abnormal Child Psychology*, 28, 467-479.

doi:10.1300/J005v33n01_05

HIV Prevention Services for Adults with Serious Mental Illness in Public Mental Health Care Programs

Eric R. Wright
Dustin E. Wright
Anthony H. Lawson

Indiana University–Purdue University at Indianapolis

SUMMARY. Despite well-documented need, little is known about the HIV prevention services provided to adults with serious mental illness in the public mental health system. This study examined the types, frequency, and client-level correlates of HIV prevention services provided to a representative sample of clients in five public mental health care programs. Although results indicate that HIV prevention care is infrequent, clients identified as being at higher risk for HIV infection reported receiving prevention interventions more frequently. However, both the clients' gender and the service setting influenced the types and frequency of services that clients received. doi:10.1300/J005v33n01_06 *[Article copies available for a fee from The Haworth Document Delivery Service: 1-800-HAWORTH. E-mail address: <docdelivery@haworthpress.com>*

Address correspondence to: Eric R. Wright, Indiana University-Purdue University Indianapolis (IUPUI), Department of Sociology, 425 University Boulevard, CA 303, Indianapolis, IN 46202-5140 (E-mail: ewright@iupui.edu).

This research was supported by grants from the National Institute of Mental Health (Grant No. R01 MH59717) and from the Indiana University Research and University Graduate School.

[Haworth co-indexing entry note]: "HIV Prevention Services for Adults with Serious Mental Illness in Public Mental Health Care Programs." Wright, Eric R., Dustin E. Wright, and Anthony H. Lawson. Co-published simultaneously in *Journal of Prevention & Intervention in the Community* (The Haworth Press, Inc.) Vol. 33, No.1/2, 2007, pp. 63-77; and: *HIV: Issues with Mental Health and Illness* (ed: Michael B. Blank, and Marlene M. Eisenberg) The Haworth Press, Inc., 2007, pp. 63-77. Single or multiple copies of this article are available for a fee from The Haworth Document Delivery Service [1-800-HAWORTH, 9:00 a.m. - 5:00 p.m. (EST). E-mail address: docdelivery@haworthpress.com].

KEYWORDS. HIV prevention, people with mental illness, mental health services

Concern about the spread of HIV/AIDS among people with severe mental illness (SMI) has led many researchers and policy makers to ask what, if anything, mental health professionals are doing to respond to the expanding epidemic (Cournos, McKinnon, & Rosner, 2001; McKinnon et al., 1999; Sullivan et al., 1999). Consumers and client advocates often claim that treatment providers are reticent about discussing sexuality-related issues, including HIV transmission (Deegan, 1999). At the same time, surveys of mental health administrators suggest that public mental health agencies face significant barriers to providing HIV prevention services to their clients with SMI (Herman, Kaplan, Satriano, Cournos, & McKinnon, 1994; Knox, 1998; McKinnon et al., 1999). There is, however, little empirical data on what HIV prevention services clients with SMI are receiving in the public mental health system. Using data gathered from a representative sample of clients enrolled in five public mental health treatment programs for adults with SMI, this paper examines clients' reports of the HIV prevention services they received from their mental health care providers in order to better understand what mental health professionals are doing to respond to the HIV epidemic among adults with SMI.

Background

Despite a growing concern about the spread of HIV/AIDS among people with SMI (Cournos et al., 2001; Sullivan et al., 1999), research indicates that most clients with SMI are unlikely to receive HIV prevention services from their mental health clinicians (Coverdale & Aruffo, 1992; McKinnon et al., 1999; Walkup, Satriano, Hansell, & Olfson, 1998). Anecdotal reports indicate that mental health professionals often do not address sexuality and HIV-related issues with their clients with SMI. Advocates and consumers, for example, have complained for many years that clinicians neglect their clients' sexual needs (Deegan, 1999; Lukoff, Gioia-Hasik, Sullivan, Golden, & Nuechterlein, 1986), including their hopes and desires for developing romantic partnerships (Davidson &

Stayner, 1997; Ginsberg, 1977; Wasow, 1980) and their concerns about the sexual side-effects of psychotropic medication (Buffum, 1982; Holbrook, 1989; Kockott & Pfeiffer, 1996). Indeed, several client advocates have argued that sexuality is an "unmentionable" topic in most mental health programs (Coverdale & Aruffo, 1992; Herman et al., 1994; Rowe & Savage, 1987; Ryan, 1990; Schell, 1994).

More formal research echoes clients' concerns and provides further evidence that mental health professionals are not consistently assessing or intervening with clients' HIV-related needs (Coverdale & Aruffo, 1992; Hellerstein & Prager, 1992; Herman et al., 1994; Mitchell, Grindel, & Laurenzano, 1996; Ryan, 1990; Walkup et al., 1998). Several studies have found that general hospital psychiatric staff often fail to identify clients with significant HIV risk or histories of serious sexual abuse and dysfunction (Hellerstein & Prager, 1992; Mitchell et al., 1996; Walkup et al., 1998). Coverdale and Aruffo (1992) surveyed community mental health professionals and found that "nearly all" reported that clients should be counseled about HIV/AIDS and family planning but that only 20-25% of their patients actually received such information. While these studies infer that many mental health professionals may be uncomfortable talking about sexuality and HIV with their clients, there is some indication that this is changing. In a recent survey, Walkup and colleagues (1998) found that of 53 psychiatric units in New York State, only 9 percent reported that they did nothing to educate or counsel clients about HIV. Nevertheless, McKinnon et al. (1999), based on data gathered from a large sample of mental health administrators, reported that treatment agencies face significant barriers to providing effective HIV prevention services to their clients, including lack of funds to pay for condoms and inadequately trained staff.

At the same time, there are a number of published reports of mental health professionals' efforts to respond to the HIV-related needs of clients with serious mental illness (Carmen & Brady, 1990; Cournos, Empfield, Horwath, & Kramer, 1989; Knox, 1989). A review of this literature reveals four general groups of HIV prevention interventions used by mental health professionals with adult clients with SMI. First, many institutions and some community-based programs have used *restrictions* to manage clients' disruptive sexual behavior. Typically, this has involved the use of seclusion rooms, physical restraints, and/or one-on-one staff supervision to limit clients' abilities to put themselves or others at risk (Ginsberg, 1977; Holbrook, 1989; Wasow, 1980). However, they also may include less tangible forms of restrictiveness, such as restricting clients' sexual and risk-taking autonomy (Bachrach, 1980; Carpenter, 1978;

Garritson, 1987; Munertz & Geller, 1993). Second, mental health professionals have offered clients basic *HIV prevention education*. Because of the special cognitive difficulties associated with SMI, mental health professionals have relied on specialized curricula (Cates, Bond, & Graham, 1994; Goisman, Kent, Montgomery, Cheevers, & Goldfinger, 1991; Lauer-Listhaus & Watterson, 1988; Lewis & Scott, 1997; Lukoff, Sullivan, & Goisman, 1992; Schindler & Ferguson, 1995; Sladyk, 1990). These programs typically involve providing clients with brochures about the "facts" of HIV or safer sex (usually when clients ask about HIV or AIDS) or inviting clients to participate in voluntary sexuality or HIV discussion or education groups. Third, mental health providers have tried to *integrate HIV-related issues into standard psychotherapy and case management* for mental illness clients. Several therapeutic assessment and intervention models targeting various risk behaviors have been proposed for clinicians who do psychotherapy and/or case management with clients with SMI (Friedrich & Grannan, 1998; Knox, 1989; Knox, 1998). Counseling has been shown to be a particularly effective forum for dealing with clients' sexual dysfunction, the sexual side-effects of medications, working through difficulties in maintaining sexual and/or romantic relationships, and addressing "co-factors" or issues which often reinforce high risk behavior, including substance use and self-esteem problems (Buffum, 1982; Kockott & Pfeiffer, 1996; Savin-Williams & Lenhart, 1990; Vincke, Bolton, Mak, & Blank, 1993). Fourth, and most recently, several clinical research groups have proposed and tested *HIV prevention skills training and support* programs (Carey et al., 2004; Kalichman, Sikkema, Kelly, & Bulto, 1995; Kaplan & Herman, 1996; Otto-Salaj, Kelly, Stevenson, Hoffman, & Kalichman, 2001; Otto-Salaj, Stevenson, & Kelly, 1996; Susser et al., 1998). In these models, small groups of people with SMI are provided basic information about HIV, its transmission, and various risk behaviors over a series of group and/or individual sessions, while also being given the opportunity to develop specific skills to implement risk reduction strategies.

While these general models offer some clinical guidance for addressing clients' HIV-related needs, the research on these intervention strategies is limited to small exploratory or efficacy studies of particular approaches conducted under well-controlled conditions. More important, because the emphasis has been on developing intervention protocols, we know very little about what HIV prevention services mental health professionals are actually providing in their daily practice. The purpose of this study was to describe and examine the client-level correlates of the HIV-related prevention services provided to adults with SMI in public mental health care programs.

METHOD

The data for this study come from the Indiana Mental Health Services and HIV Risk Study. As part of this study, face-to-face interviews were conducted with clients in treatment programs for individuals with SMI at three community mental health centers (CMHCs) and two state psychiatric hospitals. Clients who met the following criteria were invited to participate: (1) a diagnosis of a SMI (e.g., schizophrenia or schizophrenia-spectrum disorders, bipolar disorder, major depression, or other major mental disorder, involving psychosis or imposing major limitations on daily functioning); (2) a psychiatric treatment history of two years or longer; (3) enrolled for treatment at the field site for at least three months; (4) not currently subject to criminal charges or residing in jail; and, (5) between the ages of 18 and 55. The final sample included 401 clients across the five facilities. The overall client participation rate was 74%. A number of clients were unable to complete the entire interview for a variety of reasons, including the section of the interview related to the HIV-related prevention services. These 32 clients were not included in this study, resulting in a final analysis sample of 369 clients.

The study interview protocol contained a standardized self-report tool (Wright & Wright, 2004) for measuring how often clients believed they received specific HIV-related prevention mental health services, and how often they believed they had talked about sexuality or HIV-related issues with the most important members of their treatment team. The items measuring HIV-related prevention services were developed by the first author for this study based on interventions reported in the published literature. Individual items asked clients to indicate how frequently they had received various services or therapeutic recommendations from the four major theoretical groups of HIV-related prevention mental health services: therapeutic restrictions, HIV prevention education, HIV-focused psychotherapy and case management, and HIV prevention skills training and support. Clients replied using a 4-point scale (0 = "never"; 1 = "once or twice"; 2 = "several times"; 3 = "frequently") to indicate the frequency at which they received each of the interventions.

Several demographic (i.e., gender, age, race, sexual identity, marital status, education, recent sexual activity) and clinical variables (i.e., diagnosis, global assessment of functioning [GAF] score, number of prior hospitalizations, HIV sero-status) were included in this study to both describe the sample and for use as controls in the multivariate analyses. HIV sero-status, psychiatric diagnosis, and GAF scores were collected from enrolled clients' clinical records and medical charts. In the multivariate analyses, we used dummy variables to indicate the three most common primary diagnoses (i.e., schizophrenia/schizophrenia-spectrum disorders, bipolar disorder, and major depression with and without psychotic features), so all "other diagnoses" served as the reference category. To identify those clients who were currently sexually active, we used a dummy variable to indicate those clients who reported having had one or more sexual partners during the preceding three months.

RESULTS

Description of Services Provided

Table 1 displays descriptive statistics and psychometrics for the total sample for each service category subscale, as well as a comparison of the hospital and CMHC samples. The most frequently provided category of service was HIV prevention education ($M = 0.50$, $SD = 0.65$). The least frequent category of services received were HIV prevention skills ($M = 0.34$, $SD = 0.50$) and therapeutic restrictions ($M = 0.37$, $SD = 0.57$). Each subscale was factor analyzed to assess the unidimensionality of the subscale. As shown in Table 1, a one-factor model of each subscale explained at least 41% of the variance. Additionally, each subscale displayed good internal validity, with alpha coefficients ranging from .76 to .88.

Service Setting Analyses

In order to describe the differences in HIV-related service provision between state hospitals and CMHCs, a series of one-way ANOVAs were computed to test for differences between service sites. Clients in state hospitals ($M = 0.53$, $SD = 0.64$) reported receiving therapeutic restrictions significantly more frequently than clients in CMHCs ($M = 0.24$, $SD = 0.47$, $F (1, 367) = 25.06$, $p < .001$). Additionally, service provision between each state hospital and each CMHC was compared. State hospital 2 was significantly more likely to have provided HIV-related education services ($M = 0.66$, $SD = 0.67$) than state hospital 1 ($M = 0.41$, $SD = 0.55$, $F (2, 167) = 7.00$, $p < .01$). Likewise, a significant difference was observed be-

TABLE 1. Frequency of HIV-Prevention Services by Service Site

	Therapeutic Restrictions M (SD)	HIV Prevention Education M (SD)	HIV-Focused Counseling & Case Management M (SD)	HIV Prevention Skills Training & Support M (SD)
State Hospitals (N = 169)	0.53 (0.64)	0.54 (0.63)	0.46 (0.60)	0.33 (0.48)
1 (N = 81)	0.49 (0.57)	0.41 (0.55)	0.37 (0.49)	0.24 (0.39)
2 (N = 88)	0.56 (0.70)	0.66 (0.67)	0.54 (0.68)	0.41 (0.55)
F (1, 167)	0.49	7.00**	3.51	5.01*
CMHCs (N = 200)	0.24 (0.47)	0.47 (0.67)	0.49 (0.62)	0.34 (0.51)
1 (N = 70)	0.24 (0.42)	0.57 (0.76)	0.59 (0.68)	0.36 (0.48)
2 (N = 72)	0.11 (0.29)	0.33 (0.55)	0.37 (0.48)	0.25 (0.41)
3 (N = 58)	0.41 (0.62)	0.53 (0.66)	0.51 (0.70)	0.44 (0.63)
F (2, 197)	7.12***	2.68	2.26	2.31
TOTAL (N = 369)	0.37 (0.57)	0.50 (0.65)	0.47 (0.61)	0.34 (0.50)
F (1, 367)	25.06***	0.99	0.16	.011
Eigenvalue	2.80	4.82	3.44	2.89
% of Variance Explained	46.73	53.51	49.12	41.29
Alpha	0.77	0.88	0.82	0.76

Post-hoc Scheffé analysis revealed a significant difference between CMHCs 2 & 3 on the Therapeutic Restrictions Index, $p < .001$.
*$p < .05$. **$p < .01$. ***$p < .001$.

tween CMHCs, with clients at CMHC 3 reporting that they received significantly more therapeutic restrictions ($M = 0.41, SD = 0.62$) than clients at CMHC 2 ($M = 0.11, SD = 0.29, F(2, 197) = 7.12, p < .001$) as confirmed by a post-hoc Scheffé analysis.

Regression Analyses–Predictors of Frequency of Service Provision

A series of OLS regressions was performed in order to describe a model of the frequency of service provision for each of the categories of HIV-related mental health services. Each of these models included a set of demographic and clinical variables as well as dummy variables for each of the sites included in this study. OLS regressions using a "hospital v. CMHC" dummy variable were also performed, although those models did not account for as much of the variance as the models in which each site was included separately (details available upon request). Furthermore, the individual sites were frequently significant predictors in the model, implying that the effect of treatment environment is better captured when indicators for the individual sites were used. The dependent variable for each model was the average frequency at which clients reported having received the services in each service category.

Table 2 presents the results of the OLS regressions for each category of HIV-related mental health service. The model for therapeutic restrictions was significant ($F = 3.95, p < .001$) and explained 15% of the variance in how frequently clients reported receiving therapeutic restrictions. Clients who were HIV positive ($\beta = .11$) and sexually active in the preceding three months ($\beta = .18$) were significantly more likely to report staff recommending or applying therapeutic restrictions. Clients receiving services at CMHC 1 ($\beta = -.20$) and CMHC 2 ($\beta = -.28$) were significantly less likely to report the use of therapeutic restrictions.

The model for HIV prevention education was significant ($F = 2.94, p < .001$) and explained 12% of the variance in how frequently clients reported receiving HIV prevention education services. In this model, we found that women clients reported receiving significantly less HIV prevention education than men. Similar to the previous model, HIV positive status ($\beta = .11$) and being currently sexually active ($\beta = .15$) were associated with receiving HIV prevention education services significantly more frequently. Clients at Hospital 2 were also significantly more likely to report receiving more frequent HIV prevention services ($\beta = .20$) than clients in Hospital 1, indicating that HIV prevention at Hospital 2 was provided at levels similar to those found in the three CMHCs.

The model for HIV-focused counseling and case management was significant ($F = 2.19, p < .01$) and explained 9% of the variance in how frequently clients reported receiving HIV-focused counseling and case management services. The clients most likely to receive this type of service were those who were currently sexually active ($\beta = .18$) and those receiving services at Hospital 2 ($\beta = .14$).

Finally, the model for HIV prevention skills training and support was also significant ($F = 1.88, p < .05$), explaining 8% of the variance in how frequently clients reported receiving HIV prevention skills training ser-

TABLE 2. Regression Analyses of HIV-Prevention Services (N = 369)

Variable	Therapeutic Restrictions			HIV Prevention Education			HIV-Focused Counseling & Case Management			HIV Prevention Skills Training & Support		
	B	SEB	β	B	SEB	β	B	SEB	β	B	SEB	β
Constant	.28	.18		.15	.21		.10	.20		.13	.16	
Age	.00	.00	.02	.00	.00	−.04	.00	.00	−.01	.00	.00	−.02
Race (Non-white)	.01	.06	.01	.12	.07	.09	.11	.07	.09	.06	.06	.06
Gender (Female)	−.11	.06	−.10	−.22	.07	−.17***	−.11	.07	−.09	−.12	.0	−.12*
Marital Status (Married or Cohabitating)	−.09	.10	−.05	.02	.12	−.01	−.12	.11	−.06	−.10	.09	−.06
Sexual Orientation (Homosexuality)	.14	.09	.07	.07	.11	.03	.10	.11	.05	−.05	.09	−.03
Schizophrenia	.04	.08	.03	.07	.10	.05	.00	.09	.00	.04	.07	.04
Depression	−.05	.12	−.02	.05	.14	.02	.04	.13	.02	−.01	.11	−.01
Bipolar Disorder	.17	.20	.05	.12	.23	.03	.19	.22	.05	−.01	.18	.00
# of Hospitalizations	.01	.01	.05	.02	.01	.07	.01	.01	.07	.02	.01	.10
GAF Score	.00	.00	.05	.01	.00	.10	.00	.00	.09	.00	.00	.02
HIV Positive	.42	.20	.11*	.50	.23	.11*	.37	.22	.09	.30	.18	.09
Sexually Active in past 3 months	.22	.07	.18***	.20	.08	.15**	.24	.07	.18***	.14	.06	.13*
Hospital 2[a]	.07	.09	.05	.31	.10	.20**	.21	.10	.14*	.19	.08	.16*
CMHC 1 [a]	−.29	.11	−.20**	.16	.13	.10	.18	.12	.11	.16	.10	.12
CMHC 2 [a]	−.40	.10	−.28***	−.11	.12	−.06	−.04	.11	−.03	.03	.09	.02
CMHC 3 [a]	−.06	.10	−.04	.19	.11	.11	.17	.11	.10	.25	.09	.18**
F	3.95***			2.94***			2.19**			1.88*		
S.E.E.	.54			.63			.60			.49		
R Square	.15			.12			.09			.08		

[a] Hospital 1 is reference category.
*p < .05. **p < .01. ***p < .001.

vices. In this model, we found that being a woman client significantly decreased the likelihood of receiving HIV prevention skills training and support. Being currently sexually active ($\beta = .13$) and in treatment at Hospital 2 ($\beta = .16$) and CMHC 3 ($\beta = .18$), however, were associated with a significant increase in the frequency of reporting HIV prevention skills training and support.

DISCUSSION

The purpose of this study was to empirically examine the HIV prevention-related mental health services clients in hospital and community-based care are receiving. We found that clients reported receiving very few HIV prevention-related mental health services. Indeed, in most cases, less than one third of the clients we surveyed said that they had received any of the prevention services included in our list of interventions. This finding is similar to other published reports that found low rates of HIV prevention-related mental health services based on surveys of mental health administrators and clinical staff (McKinnon et al., 1999; Walkup et al., 1998; Wright & Martin, 2003). In this regard, our findings validate mental health administrators' and clinicians' impressions at the client-level.

Our findings further indicate that HIV prevention skills training–the most intensive class of services–was the type of care least likely to be provided to the clients we surveyed. The use of therapeutic restrictions to manage high-risk behavior also was infrequent, possibly reflecting more open attitudes about client sexuality in the mental health system. In general, the clients we surveyed reported receiving HIV prevention education and HIV-related therapy or counseling most frequently. While clinical decision-making is a complex process influenced by many factors, our study suggests that when professionals in public mental health try to provide HIV preventive care, they tend to emphasize services that require less training and skill, as well as interventions that are more easily integrated into traditional psychiatric treatment models. The relatively low frequency of HIV-related skills training is particularly important, however, because these methods reflect the only class of interventions for which there is some demonstrated efficacy in reducing clients' HIV risk behavior (Carey et al., 2004; Kalichman et al., 1995; Otto-Salaj et al., 2001; Susser et al., 1998).

The results of our multiple regression analyses further highlight that HIV prevention-related services were provided most frequently to a small sub-set of clients. Specifically, those clients who were known to be HIV positive, currently sexually active, and more acutely mentally ill (i.e., hospitalized) were the clients most likely to report receiving more of all four types of care. It appears that staff may be intentionally targeting the highest risk clients for HIV prevention-related interventions. Unfortunately, the cross-sectional nature of our data makes it impossible to know exactly why this pattern exists. It may be that these individual-level characteristics are influencing staff perceptions of need and/or clinical decision-making. However, it also may be that clients who fit this profile are simply more likely to raise these issues with staff and request support and services from their care providers.

At the same time, the concentration of services within this sub-group of consumers also means that, because of the low-prevalence of these characteristics in client populations, most clients who are not currently at risk are significantly less likely to receive HIV prevention-related mental health services. While this pattern may not have immediate consequences for the spread of HIV, it may reflect a general reactive bias among mental health professionals when it comes to providing this type of care. That is, rather than addressing these issues proactively with clients who have the potential for engaging in high risk behavior, clinicians may assume that clients are generally not at risk and/or rely on clients to bring up these special concerns before considering or assessing clients' needs for HIV prevention services.

Overall, few demographic predictors of HIV-related service provision were found, suggesting that the provision of these services is evenly distributed to a broad range of clients. One notable exception to this pattern was with regard to gender, where women reported receiving significantly fewer instances of HIV-related prevention education or HIV-related skills training than men, even after controlling for current sexual activity. We believe this pattern may reflect broader societal beliefs and assumptions regarding women's sexuality, such that mental health professionals may be more prone to overlook or ignore the HIV prevention needs of women in their care.

Finally, we also found variation in the patterns of HIV prevention-related mental health services provision to clients across the five sites we studied, primarily in the use of therapeutic restrictions. Overall, hospitals were more likely to emphasize therapeutic restrictions than CMHCs. However, even among the CMHCs there was significant variability in the use of therapeutic restrictions. The two sites where this type of care was less frequent were somewhat different from the third CMHC because they had a stronger organizational commitment to providing services within a psychosocial rehabilitation framework and because they provided more integrated residential care (e.g., semi-independent living program, cluster apartments) rather than traditional group home care. Conversely, the CMHC that used therapeutic restrictions more frequently relied more extensively on group homes for providing residential care, including several "secure facilities."

Two other site-specific differences were observed. Clients at CMHC 3 were significantly more likely to report more frequent HIV prevention skills training and support. Although it is difficult to know precisely why, informal ethnographic observations made during the implementation of the larger study revealed that this site had a particularly strong day treatment program that emphasized skills-training in a variety of areas, including interpersonal relationships and sexuality. The manager of this program, as well as many staff, also mentioned that they had had formal training in sex education. It is unclear, however, why the unique attitudes and beliefs of staff in this treatment setting did not also result in significantly higher rates of HIV prevention education and HIV-related therapy and case management.

In addition, receiving services at Hospital 2 was a significant predictor of receiving almost all HIV-related mental health services more frequently. As with CMHC 3, a number of organizationally-specific characteristics may explain this finding. Hospital 2 had a reputation among patients of being more supportive and tolerant of patient sexual expression than the other hospital where this study was conducted. In fact, several subjects in our study who had been admitted to both hospitals over the years commented on how much "easier" it was to have sex at Hospital 2 than Hospital 1, and several subjects even mentioned significant others they had "waiting" for them at Hospital 2. Similarly, the front-line staff at Hospital 2, primarily psychiatric attendants, assumed much of the responsibility for providing sexuality and HIV-related services to clients and passively-accepted patient-to-patient romantic relationships. Conversely, policy at Hospital 1 explicitly dictated that sex education and counseling was the exclusive responsibility of the professional staff (e.g., psychiatrists, nurses, etc.) and that patients were not allowed, under any circumstances, to have sexual contact with each other. Regardless of the unique qualities of the five sites, it is clear that these differences go beyond the type of care provided (e.g., hospital v. community care). Rather, we believe that these differences point to the importance of the organizational culture of facilities as an important determinant of the provision of HIV prevention services within mental health care programs (Wright, 2001).

CONCLUSION

In conclusion, our study found that HIV prevention-related mental health services are a relatively infrequent feature of treatment for adult clients with SMI in the public mental health system. This was especially true of the more intensive and effective evidence-based services involving prevention skills training. Nevertheless, we did find that clients who reported having the greatest current level of HIV-risk were significantly more likely to say they had received these services than other clients, although there also was evidence that women clients, regardless of their risk level, were less likely to receive even basic HIV prevention education and HIV-related therapy and case management. More important, we also found that there was significant variation in the frequency and type of HIV prevention services provided to this population across different mental health service settings. Taken together, our findings underline the need to examine more carefully the role of mental health professionals and psychiatric treatment in addressing the HIV prevention needs of adults with SMI.

REFERENCES

Bachrach, L. L. (1980). Is the least restrictive environment always the best? Sociological and semantic implications. *Hospital and Community Psychiatry, 31*(2), 97-103.

Buffum, J. (1982). Pharmacosexology: The effects of drugs on sexual function: A review. *Journal of Psychoactive Drugs, 14*(1-2), 5-44.

Carey, M. P., Carey, K. B., Maisto, S. A., Gordon, C. M., Schroder, K. E. E., & Vanable, P. A. (2004). Reducing HIV-risk behavior among adults receiving outpatient psychiatric treatment: Results from a randomized controlled trial. *Journal of Consulting and Clinical Psychology, 72*(2), 252-268.

Carmen, E., & Brady, S. M. (1990). AIDS risk and prevention for the chronic mentally ill. *Hospital and Community Psychiatry, 41*(6), 652-657.

Carpenter, M. D. (1978). Residential placement for the chronic psychiatric patient: A review and evaluation of the literature. *Schizophrenia Bulletin, 4*(3), 384-98.

Cates, J. A., Bond, G. R., & Graham, L. L. (1994). AIDS knowledge, attitudes, and risk behavior among people with serious mental illness. *Psychosocial Rehabilitation Journal, 17*(4), 19-29.

Cournos, F., Empfield, M., Horwath, E., & Kramer, M. (1989). The management of HIV infection in state hospitals. *Hospital and Community Psychiatry, 40*(2), 153-57.

Cournos, F., McKinnon, K., & Rosner, J. (2001). HIV among individuals with severe mental illness. *Psychiatric Annals, 31*(1), 50-56.

Coverdale, J. H., & Aruffo, J. F. (1992). AIDS and family planning counseling of psychiatrically ill women in community mental health clinics. *Community Mental Health Journal, 28*(1), 13-20.

Davidson, L., & Stayner, D. (1997). Loss, loneliness, and the desire for love: Perspectives on the social lives of people with schizophrenia. *Psychiatric Rehabilitation Journal, 20*(3), 3-12.

Deegan, P. E. (1999). Human sexuality and mental illness: Consumer viewpoints and recovery principles. In P. F. Buckley (Ed.), *Sexuality and Serious Mental Illness* (pp. 21-34). Amsterdam, The Netherlands: Harwood Academic Publishers.

Friedrich, M. A., & Grannan, J. A. (1998). Treating persons with serious and persistent mental illness. In M. Knox & C. H. Sparks (Eds.), *HIV and Community Mental Health Care* (pp. 250-265). Baltimore, MD: Johns Hopkins University Press.

Garritson, S. H. (1987). Characteristics of restrictiveness. *Journal of Psychosocial Nursing and Mental Health Services, 25*(1), 10-19.

Ginsberg, L. H. (1977). The institutionalized mentally disabled. In H. L. Gochros & J. S. Gochros (Eds.), *The Sexually Oppressed* (pp. 215-224). New York, NY: Association Press.

Goisman, R. M., Kent, A. B., Montgomery, E. C., Cheevers, M. M., & Goldfinger, S. M. (1991). AIDS education for patients with chronic mental illness. *Community Mental Health Journal, 27*(3), 189-197.

Hellerstein, D. J., & Prager, M. E. (1992). Assessing HIV risk in the general hospital psychiatric clinic. *General Hospital Psychiatry, 14,* 3-6.

Herman, R., Kaplan, M., Satriano, J., Cournos, F., & McKinnon, K. (1994). HIV prevention with persons with serious mental illness: Staff training and institutional attitudes. *Psychosocial Rehabilitation Journal, 17*(4), 97-104.

Holbrook, T. (1989). Policing sexuality in a modern state hospital. *Hospital and Community Psychiatry, 40*(1), 75-79.

Kalichman, S. C., Sikkema, K. J., Kelly, J. A., & Bulto, M. (1995). Use of a brief behavioral skills intervention to prevent HIV infection among chronic mentally ill adults. *Psychiatric Services, 46*(3), 275-280.

Kaplan, M., & Herman, R. (1996). Cognitive-behavioral risk reduction groups for teaching safer sex. In F. Cournos & N. Bakalar (Eds.), *AIDS and People with Serious Mental Illness* (pp. 125-135). New Haven, CT: Yale University Press.

Knox, M. D. (1989). Community mental health's role in the AIDS crisis. *Community Mental Health Journal, 25*(3), 185-196.

Knox, M. D. (1998). HIV-related community mental health services. In M. Knox & C. H. Sparks (Eds.), *HIV and Community Mental Health Care* (pp. 3-16). Baltimore, MD: Johns Hopkins University Press.

Kockott, G., & Pfeiffer, W. (1996). Sexual disorders in nonacute psychiatric outpatients. *Comprehensive Psychiatry, 37*(1), 56-61.

Lauer-Listhaus, B., & Watterson, J. (1988). A psychoeducational group for HIV-positive patients on a psychiatric service. *Hospital and Community Psychiatry, 39*(7), 776-77.

Lewis, J., & Scott, E. (1997). The sexual education needs of those disabled by mental illness. *Psychiatric Rehabilitation Journal, 21*(2), 164-167.

Lukoff, D., Gioia-Hasik, D., Sullivan, G., Golden, J. S., & Nuechterlein, K. H. (1986). Sex education and rehabilitation with schizophrenic male outpatients. *Schizophrenia Bulletin, 12*(4), 669-766.

Lukoff, D., Sullivan, J. G., & Goisman, R. M. (1992). Sex and AIDS education. In R. P. Liberman (Ed.), *Handbook of Psychiatric Rehabilitation* (pp. 171-182). New York, NY: Macmillan Publishing Company.

McKinnon, K., Cournos, F., Herman, R., Satriano, J., Silver, B. J., & Puello, I. (1999). AIDS-related services and training in outpatient mental health care agencies in New York. *Psychiatric Services, 50*(9), 1225-1228.

Mitchell, D., Grindel, C. G., & Laurenzano, C. (1996). Sexual abuse assessment on admission by nursing staff in general hospital psychiatric settings. *Psychiatric Services, 47*(2), 159-164.

Munertz, M. R., & Geller, J. L. (1993). The least restrictive alternative in the post-institutional era. *Hospital and Community Psychiatry, 44*(10), 967-973.

Otto-Salaj, L. L., Kelly, J. A., Stevenson, L. Y., Hoffman, R., & Kalichman, S. C. (2001). Outcomes of a randomized small-group HIV prevention trial for people with serious mental illness. *Community Mental Health Journal, 37*, 123-144.

Otto-Salaj, L. L., Stevenson, L. Y., & Kelly, J. A. (1996). Risk reduction strategies. In F. Cournos & N. Bakalar (Eds.), *AIDS and People with Serious Mental Illness* (pp. 113-124). New Haven, CT: Yale University Press.

Rowe, W. S., & Savage, S. (1987). *Sexuality and the Developmentally Handicapped.* Lewiston, NY: Edwin Mellen Press.

Ryan, C. C. (1990). The training and support of health care professionals dealing with the psychiatric aspects of AIDS. In D. G. Ostrow (Ed.), *Behavioral Aspects of AIDS* (pp. 355-392). New York, NY: Plenum Press.

Savin-Williams, R. C., & Lenhart, R. E. (1990). AIDS prevention among gay and lesbian youth: Psychosocial stress and health care intervention guidelines. In D. G. Ostrow (Ed.), *Behavioral Aspects of AIDS* (pp. 75-99). New York, NY: Plenum Press.

Schell, B. H. (1994). The unmentionable. *The Journal of the California Alliance for the Mentally Ill, 5*(2), 58-60.

Schindler, V., & Ferguson, S. (1995). An educational program on acquired immunodeficiency syndrome for patients with mental illness. *American Journal of Occupational Therapy, 49*(4), 359-361.

Sladyk, K. (1990). Teaching safe sex practices to psychiatric patients. *American Journal of Occupational Therapy, 44*(3), 284-286.

Sullivan, G., Koegel, P., Kanouse, D. E., Cournos, F., McKinnon, K., Young, A. et al. (1999). HIV and people with serious mental illness: The public sector's role in reducing HIV risk and improving care. *Psychiatric Services, 50*(5), 648-652.

Susser, E., Valencia, E., Berkman, A., Sohler, N., Conover, S., Torres, J. et al. (1998). Human immunodeficiency virus sexual risk reduction in homeless men with mental illness. *Archives of General Psychiatry, 55*, 266-272.

Vincke, J., Bolton, R., Mak, R., & Blank, S. (1993). Coming out and AIDS-related high-risk sexual behavior. *Archives of Sexual Behavior, 22*(6), 559-586.

Walkup, J., Satriano, J., Hansell, S., & Olfson, M. (1998). Practices related to HIV risk assessment in general hospital psychiatric units in New York State. *Psychiatric Services, 49*(4), 529-530.

Wasow, M. (1980). Sexuality and the institutionalized mentally ill. *Sexuality and Disability, 3*(1), 3-16.

Wright, D. E., & Wright, E. R. (2004). *The HIV Prevention-Related Mental Health Services Scale.* Indiana University-Purdue University Indianapolis, Applied Medical Social Science Web site: http://www.amss.iupui.edu.

Wright, E. R., & Martin, T. N. (2003). The social organization of HIV/AIDS care in treatment programs for adults with serious mental illness. *AIDS Care, 15*(6), 763-773.

doi:10.1300/J005v33n01_06

Differences in HIV-Related Knowledge, Attitudes, and Behavior Among Psychiatric Outpatients With and Without a History of a Sexually Transmitted Infection

Peter A. Vanable

Michael P. Carey

Kate B. Carey

Stephen A. Maisto

Syracuse University

SUMMARY. HIV infection among the mentally ill is estimated to be at least eight times the prevalence in the general population. Psychiatric patients may also be disproportionately vulnerable to other sexually transmitted infections (STIs), but this has not been well studied. We sought to characterize the prevalence and correlates of STIs in a sample

Address correspondence to: Peter A. Vanable, Assistant Professor, Center for Health and Behavior, 430 Huntington Hall, Syracuse University, Syracuse, NY 13244.

The authors thank Brian Borsari, Susan Collins, Christopher Correia, Lauren Durant, Julie Fuller, Christopher Gordon, John Harkulich, JulieAnn Hartley, Vardit Konsens, Dan Neal, Teal Pedlow, Mary Beth Pray, Daniel Purnine, Kerstin Schroder, Jeffrey Simons, Lance Weinhardt, Adrienne Williams, Emily Wright, and Denise Zona for their assistance with the project.

This work was supported by the National Institute of Mental Health Grants R01-MH54929 and R21-MH65865.

[Haworth co-indexing entry note]: "Differences in HIV-Related Knowledge, Attitudes, and Behavior Among Psychiatric Outpatients With and Without a History of a Sexually Transmitted Infection." Vanable, Peter A. et al. Co-published simultaneously in *Journal of Prevention & Intervention in the Community* (The Haworth Press, Inc.) Vol. 33, No.1/2, 2007, pp. 79-94; and: *HIV: Issues with Mental Health and Illness* (ed: Michael B. Blank, and Marlene M. Eisenberg) The Haworth Press, Inc., 2007, pp. 79-94. Single or multiple copies of this article are available for a fee from The Haworth Document Delivery Service [1-800-HAWORTH, 9:00 a.m. - 5:00 p.m. (EST). E-mail address: docdelivery@haworthpress.com].

79

of psychiatric outpatients ($N = 464$). Over one-third of the sample (38%) reported a lifetime history of one or more STIs. Multivariate analyses showed that, relative to those without an STI history, patients with a lifetime STI history were more knowledgeable about HIV, expressed stronger intentions to use condoms, and perceived themselves to be at greater risk for HIV. However, those with a past STI were also more likely to report sex with multiple partners and reported more frequent unprotected sex in the past 3 months. Treatment for an STI may increase HIV knowledge and risk reduction motivation, but does not necessarily lead to changes in sexual risk behavior among psychiatric patients. Findings highlight the need for STI/HIV risk reduction interventions in psychiatric settings, particularly for patients with high-risk profiles. doi:10.1300/J005v33n01_07   *[Article copies available for a fee from The Haworth Document Delivery Service: 1-800-HAWORTH. E-mail address: <docdelivery@haworthpress.com> Website: <http://www.HaworthPress.com> © 2007 by The Haworth Press, Inc. All rights reserved.]*

KEYWORDS. HIV-related knowledge, sexually transmitted infections, risk behaviors, serious mental illness

The prevalence of HIV infection among people living with a mental illness is as much as eight times the prevalence in the general population (Carey, Weinhardt, & Carey, 1995; Rosenberg et al., 2001). Research on HIV infection among psychiatric patients has typically focused on individuals experiencing chronic and pervasive impairment in function related to a major mood disorder (i.e., depression and bipolar disorder) or a schizophrenia-spectrum disorder. Across these disorders, psychiatric symptoms, stigma, and other life challenges may reduce the salience of non-mental (i.e., somatic) health concerns, including HIV (Carey, Carey, Weinhardt, & Gordon, 1997; Kalichman, Kelly, Johnson, & Bulto, 1994). Further, because of cognitive, social skills, and problem solving deficits, many patients with mental illness lack the requisite skills needed to negotiate safer sex (Carey et al., 1997; Gordon, Carey, Carey, Maisto, & Weinhardt, 1999; Kelly et al., 1995). Indirect factors, including the co-occurrence of substance use disorders, high levels of poverty and homelessness, and the intermingling of sexual activity within risky sexual networks, may also account for elevated risk for HIV among the mentally ill (Carey, Carey, Maisto, Gordon, & Vanable, 2001; McKinnon, Cournos, & Herman, 2001; Otto-Salaj, Heckman, Stevenson, & Kelly, 1998).

Few studies address the occurrence of STIs other than HIV among the mentally ill. Indeed, psychosocial, behavioral, and environmental factors that underlie elevated rates of HIV among the mentally ill are likely to confer increased risk for many other STIs. Recent findings from a multisite study of patients receiving care for a severe mental illness confirm that STIs other than HIV are a major health concern (Rosenberg et al., 2001). Across seven psychiatric clinics in four U.S. states ($N = 931$), 31% of patients reported a lifetime history of an STI. Further, the observed seroprevalence rates of hepatitis B (23%) and C (20%) were approximately 5 and 11 times the overall estimated population rates for these STIs respectively. Mirroring these findings, results from an STI screening study indicated that 20% of patients seen for emergency psychiatric care tested positive for a non HIV-related STI (Sitzman, Burch, Bartlett, & Urrutia, 1995). Studies conducted in STI treatment settings also point to high rates of psychopathology. For example, among 201 consecutive patients seen for STI care in a publicly funded STI clinic, 45% met criteria for an Axis I disorder as determined by a structured clinical interview (Erbelding, Hutton, Zenilman, Hunt, & Lyketsos, 2004).

Thus, initial findings highlight that STIs other than HIV are an under-recognized health concern within psychiatric settings. In the U.S., an estimated 15 million people become infected with an STI each year (Cates, 1999). Often referred to as a "hidden epidemic," many people remain unaware of the broad impact and serious health consequences of STIs (IOM, 1997). When left untreated, commonly occurring STIs can lead to severe, long term health problems, including infertility, complications during pregnancy, and several forms of life-threatening cancer. Untreated STIs also enhance a person's susceptibility to HIV infection, further highlighting the importance of early STI detection and treatment. Research that characterizes the prevalence and correlates of STIs among vulnerable subpopulations–including people with mental illness–is of considerable importance because it helps to inform prevention efforts and guide policy recommendations.

We sought to characterize the prevalence and correlates of lifetime STIs in a sample of sexually active psychiatric outpatients. We first present data on demographic, psychiatric, and substance use differences among patients with and without a lifetime STI. Next, we present data on the relationship between an STI history and current HIV-related knowledge, risk reduction motivation, and sexual risk behavior. Several studies indicate that treatment for an STI is associated with a short term reduction in sexual risk behavior (Crosby et al., 2004; Fortenberry, Brizendine, Katz, & Orr, 2002), suggesting that an STI diagnosis may serve as a "cue to action" for risk reduction. Thus, consistent with prior research and prominent conceptual formulations of sexual risk behavior (Fishbein, 2000; Fisher & Fisher, 1992; Rosenstock, Strecher, & Becker, 1994), we hypothesized that patients with a prior STI diagnosis would be sensitized to their heightened risk for HIV and, therefore, would report more favorable attitudes towards risk reduction, greater HIV knowledge, and higher levels of perceived vulnerability to HIV. We also hypothesized that participants with a past history of an STI would report fewer episodes of recent unprotected sex relative to patients without an STI history.

METHOD

Participants

Participants were recruited from two not-for-profit psychiatric hospitals for participation in a Randomized Clinical Trial (RCT) evaluating methods for reducing HIV-related risk behaviors and harmful substance use (Carey et al., 2004); the current analyses focus on data gathered during the baseline assessment. Eligibility for the RCT was limited to adult patients who were sexually active and reported alcohol or drug use in the past year. Of the 1,027 patients who met initial eligibility criteria and were recruited for the pre-intervention baseline assessment, 685 consented to participate, among whom 464 actually completed the full assessment. The mean age of participants was 37 years ($SD = 9.7$); the ethnic composition consisted of 67% White, 22% African-American, and 11% "other." Participants reported an average monthly income of less than $600 and a majority of participants (82%) were unemployed. Psychiatric diagnoses, as determined by a Structured Clinical Interview (SCID) for the DSM-IV (First, Spitzer, Gibbon, & Williams, 1995), consisted of 16% schizophrenia disorder (schizophrenia, schizophreniform disorder, or psychotic disorder NOS), 14% schizoaffective disorder, 18% bipolar disorder, 46% depressive disorder, and 7% "other." Patients reported a lifetime average of 5.9 psychiatric hospitalizations ($SD = 15.3$). Fifty nine percent of participants reported one or more episodes of unprotected vaginal or anal sex during the past 3 months.

Procedure

During standard care, a brief screening interview was used to identify patients who were sexually active and had used alcohol or recreational drugs in the previous year. Eligible patients were invited to participate in an in-depth assessment, which included a SCID interview to establish current psychiatric diagnosis, as well as a brief mental status assessment. Patients agreeing to participate in the assessment completed a detailed consent form approved by Institutional Review Boards at Syracuse University and at each hospital. To offset travel and related expenses, patients were reimbursed $30 to complete the extensive (4 to 6 hour) assessment.

Demographic, Psychiatric, and Substance Use Measures

Demographic Characteristics. Participant age, gender, marital status, ethnicity, income, educational attainment, and employment status were obtained through a structured interview.

Alcohol Use Disorders Identification Test (Saunders, Aasland, Babor, de la Fuente, & Grant, 1993). The AUDIT is a validated 10-item self-report instrument designed to identify individuals for whom the use of alcohol places them at risk for alcohol problems or who are already experiencing such problems. Summary scores range from 0-40. Prior research with persons living with a severe and persistent mental illness indicate that the AUDIT can be reliably administered and that a cut-point of 7 maximizes sensitivity and specificity scores for identifying those with an alcohol-related disorder (Maisto, Carey, Carey, Gordon, & Gleason, 2000). Coefficient alpha in the current sample was .90, providing strong evidence of measurement reliability.

Drug Abuse Screening Test (Skinner, 1982). The DAST-10 is a short version of the 28-item DAST, designed to identify drug-use related problems in the previous year. A single summary score reflects the number of drug abuse items endorsed. Research indicates that the DAST-10 is able to discriminate between psychiatric outpatients with and without current drug abuse/dependence diagnoses (Cocco & Carey, 1998). Sensitivity and specificity with this population are optimized with a score of 3 or greater (Maisto et al., 2000). Cronbach's alpha in the current sample was .83, reflecting a high degree of internal consistency.

Structured Clinical Interview for the Diagnostic and Statistical Manual of Mental Disorders (First et al., 1995). The psychotic, mood, and substance use disorders modules of the SCID-Patient Version were administered to all participants. Interviews were videotaped for the purpose of providing supervision and determining inter-rater reliability. The SCID interview typically lasted between 60 and 90 minutes, and was administered during a single session. To determine the reliability of the primary diagnoses yielded by the SCID, a second trained interviewer who was blind to diagnoses viewed a randomly sampled subset ($n = 37$) of videotapes and provided independent scoring of the SCID. There was 84% exact agreement for primary diagnosis on this subset of interviews. This agreement rate indicates a moderately high degree of reliability. SCID indices used in this study consisted of the primary Axis I psychiatric diagnosis and the clinician rated Global Assessment of Functioning (GAF) score.

Brief Symptom Inventory (Derogatis & Spencer, 1983). The BSI is a 53-item short form of the Symptom Checklist 90-Revised, an instrument designed to assess a range of psychiatric symptoms occurring within the last week. The BSI requires 10 minutes to complete; participants indicate the degree to which they were distressed by each symptom in the last week on a scale from 0 (not at all) to 4 (extremely). The Global Severity Index (GSI) derived from this self-report inventory is an index of overall symptom severity/psychological distress. In the present sample, the coefficient alpha for the global severity index (all items combined) was .97.

HIV-Related Measures

HIV Knowledge Questionnaire (Carey, Morrison, & Johnson, 1997). The HIV-KQ was used to assess knowledge related to HIV transmission and prevention. The HIV-KQ contains 45 statements and patients were asked to indicate whether the statements were true or false, or to state that they did not know. Factor analyses with diverse samples indicated that the HIV-KQ contains a single factor, is internally consistent (alpha = .91), and is stable over 2-week ($r = .91$) and 12-week ($r = .90$) intervals (Carey et al., 1997). The HIV-KQ was reliable in the current sample (alpha = .86).

Sexual Risk Reduction Motivation. Motivation was measured with 19 items that assessed condom attitudes, condom use behavioral intentions, and perceived vulnerability to HIV. *Condom attitudes* were assessed using 10 self-report items adapted from a previously validated measure (Sacco, Levine, Reed, & Thompson, 1991). Items assessing participant attitudes about condom use were rated on a 6-point Likert scale (ranging from 1 = *strongly disagree* to 6 = *strongly agree*). The coefficient alpha for the condom attitudes scale was .74. Behavioral intentions for safer sexual activities were assessed using a 6-item measure adapted from prior research with economically disadvantaged women (Carey et al., 1997). Participants were presented with a scenario describing a sexual situation, and asked to rate the likelihood of engaging in various protective behaviors (e.g., "I will tell the person that we need to practice safer sex.") and risky sexual behaviors (e.g., "I will drink or use drugs before sex.") using a six-point scale (0 = *Definitely will not do* to 5 = *Definitely will do*). Psychometric analyses indicate that the safer sex behavioral intentions measure was reliable in the current sample (alpha = .89). *Perceived risk for HIV* was measured using a 3-item scale adapted from our previous work (Carey et al., 1997). Participants rated the likelihood of contracting HIV "in the next year," and "some day." In addition, participants rated the likelihood that a "person like you" will someday get HIV. Response options ranged from "No risk at all" to "Extremely at risk." The coefficient alpha in the current sample was .89.

Sexual Risk Behavior. The time-line follow-back procedure (Carey, Carey, Maisto, Gordon, & Weinhardt, 2001) was used to assess sexual risk behavior over a 3 month interval. The TLFB involves presenting the subject with a calendar on which the target interval is marked; the sexual activity and drinking status of each day were recorded, employing strategies such as identifying extended periods of use/no use, special days (e.g., holidays), and patterned behavior. Sexual behavior outcome measures for this study consisted of a count of total number of instances of unprotected vaginal and anal sex, a measure of the proportion of sexual occasions (vaginal and anal) during which a condom was used, and a dichotomous measure indicating whether the participant reported having sex with multiple partners (yes or no), all assessed for the previous 3 months. STI history was assessed with two items that assessed the number of STIs experienced for the past year and lifetime (e.g., "In your lifetime, how many times have you had a sexually transmitted disease such as Syphilis, Gonorrhea, Herpes, or Chlamydia?").

Overview of Analyses

Statistical tests were two-tailed, and alpha was set at .05. Because the distribution of scores on the frequency measure of unprotected anal and vaginal sex was extremely skewed, frequency of unprotected sex was truncated at 105 (> 98th percentile), and the variable was then transformed using the formula ($\log_{10} X + 1$). First, descriptive analyses are presented to characterize the demographic correlates of STIs. Second, study hypotheses are tested using a series of univariate statistics to contrast psychosocial and behavioral differences among patients with and without a lifetime history of an STI. Finally, univariate correlates of STIs are included in a multivariate logistic regression analysis to characterize the independent contributions of HIV-related risk reduction information, motivation, and behavior in distinguishing patients with and without an STI history. Adjusted odds ratios and 95% confidence intervals are presented to indicate the ratio of the odds of STI status for persons with a given risk factor relative to those without the risk factor. For these analyses, categorical variables with more than two levels were recoded into dichotomous indicators using standard dummy coding procedures.

RESULTS

Prevalence and Univariate Correlates of Lifetime STIs

Over one-third of the sample (38%) reported a lifetime history of one or more STIs, and 8% reported an STI diagnosis during the previous year. Among those with a lifetime history of an STI, 52% reported that they had experienced two or more STIs ($M = 2.43$, $SD = 2.90$). Table 1 shows the demographic, substance use, and psychiatric characteristics of patients with and without a lifetime history of an STI. Patients reporting a lifetime STI were more likely to be African-American ($p < .0001$), unmarried ($p < .05$), and unemployed ($p < .05$). STI history did not vary as a function of educational attainment, gender, age, or income. As shown in Table 1, STI history did not vary as a function of psychiatric diagnosis. In addition, patients with and without a prior STI did not vary in terms of their reported level of current psychological distress or in terms of overall functional impairment as assessed by the clinician rated global assessment of functioning scale. Relative to patients with no prior STI, those reporting one or more lifetime STIs were more likely (at trend level) to screen positive for drug-related problems as assessed by the DAST (33% vs. 24%, $p < .055$), but did not differ in terms of risk for alcohol-related problems as assessed by the AUDIT.

We had hypothesized that patients with a prior STI diagnosis would report more favorable attitudes towards risk reduction, greater HIV knowledge, and higher levels of perceived vulnerability to HIV. As shown in Table 2, these hypotheses were largely confirmed. Compared to patients with no prior STIs, those with one or more lifetime STIs scored higher on the HIV knowledge questionnaire ($p < .01$), perceived themselves to be at greater risk for HIV ($p < .0001$), and reported stronger intentions to use condoms in the future ($p < .02$). Condom attitudes did not vary as a function of STI history.

Although STI history was associated with more favorable risk-reduction attitudes, an opposite trend emerged with regard to sexual risk behavior data (see Table 2). Compared to participants with no prior STIs, a

TABLE 1. Demographic, Psychiatric, and Substance Use Characteristics of Psychiatric Outpatients With and Without a Lifetime History of a Sexually Transmitted Infection (N = 464).

| | STI History | | | | | |
	Absent n = 288		Present n = 176		χ^2 (df)	p <
Demographic variables	n	%	n	%		
Gender					2.46 (1)	*ns*
Female	147	51	103	59		
Male	141	49	73	42		
Ethnicity					24.37 (4)	.0001
European-American	215	75	95	55		
African-American	42	15	58	33		
Other	30	10	21	12		
Marital status					4.49 (1)	.04
Not married	244	85	161	92		
Married	44	15	15	8		
Education					0.6 (3)	*ns*
< High school graduate	94	33	59	34		
High school graduate	94	33	62	35		
Some college	72	25	40	23		
College graduate	27	9	15	9		
Employment status					5.26 (1)	.03
Unemployed	222	77	151	86		
Employed	66	23	25	14		

	M	SD	M	SD	t (df)	p
Age	36.6	10.3	36.4	8.6	0.2 (462)	*ns*
Monthly income ($)	580	559	536	545	.81 (452)	*ns*

	n	%	n	%	χ^2 (df)	
Substance use variables						
AUDIT risk classification, %					.72 (1)	*ns*
low risk (≤ 7)	178	62	100	58		
high risk (> 7)	110	38	73	42		
DAST risk classification, %					3.75 (1)	.055
low risk (≤ 2)	217	75	118	67		
high risk (> 2)	71	25	58	33		

TABLE 1 (continued)

	Absent n = 288		Present n = 176		χ^2 (df)	p <
	n	%	n	%		
Psychiatric variables						
Diagnosis					5.10 (4)	ns
Depression	131	46	81	46		
Bipolar	55	19	27	15		
Schizophrenia	49	17	24	14		
Schizoaffective	32	11	31	18		
Other	20	7	13	7		
	M	SD	M	SD	t (df)	p
Psychological distress (BSI)	61.7	40.5	68.1	40.8	−1.63 (458)	ns
Functional impairment (GAF)	47.8	13.2	46.7	12.9	0.89 (460)	ns

Note. AUDIT = Alcohol Use Disorders Identification Test; BSI = Brief Symptom Inventory; GAF = Global Assessment of Functioning; DAST = Drug Abuse Screening Test; STI = Sexually transmitted infection.

positive STI history was associated with greater frequency of unprotected vaginal and anal sex ($p < .05$) and greater likelihood of reporting sex with multiple partners in the past 3 months ($p < .02$). The proportion of condom protected occasions of sex did not vary as a function of STI history.

Multivariate Predictors of Lifetime STIs

A hierarchical logistic regression analysis was conducted to characterize the independent contributions of HIV-related information, motivation, and sexual risk behavior in distinguishing patients with and without an STI history. Previously identified demographic correlates of STI history (marital status, employment status, and ethnicity) were entered in Step 1, followed by psychosocial and behavioral constructs identified in univariate analyses as differing as a function of STI history. Findings were largely consistent with univariate analyses. After controlling for demographic factors, HIV-related knowledge (Wald $\chi^2 = 12.2$, $p < .0001$), greater self-perceived HIV risk (Wald $\chi^2 = 9.0$, $p < .005$), and higher condom use behavioral intentions (Wald $\chi^2 = 13.2$, $p < .001$) emerged as signif-

TABLE 2. Differences in HIV-Related Knowledge, Motivation, and Risk Behavior as Function of STI History

	STI History					
	Absent (*n* = 288)		Present (*n* = 176)		*t* (df)	*p* <
Risk-behavior antecedents	M	SD	M	SD	2.73 (462)	.01
HIV Knowledge	70.9	16.0	74.9	13.9	2.73 (462)	.01
Perceived Risk for HIV	3.7	3.2	4.9	3.7	−3.83 (458)	.0001
Behavioral Intentions	20.2	7.8	22.0	7.5	−2.55 (461)	.02
Condom Attitudes	39.7	8.8	41.0	9.4	−1.53 (460)	ns
Sexual risk behavior (last 3 months)						
Number of occasions, unprotected vaginal or anal sex	9.8	18.3	14.5	25.3	−2.10 (460)	.04
Proportion of sexual occasions during which a condom was used	22.6	39.07	29.06	41.9	−1.42 (326)	ns
	n	%	*n*	%	χ^2 (df)	*p* <
Sex with multiple partners					5.97 (2)	.02
0 or 1 partners	230	80%	123	70%		
2 or more partners	58	20%	53	30%		

icant correlates of a prior STI (Model χ^2 = 40.5, p < .0001). The frequency count of unprotected vaginal and anal sex also remained as a significant predictor of STI history (Wald χ^2 = 5.01, p < .02), with higher rates of sexual risk being positively associated with a past STI diagnosis. Although sex with multiple partners and DAST scores were associated with STI history in univariate analyses, these variables did not emerge as multivariate predictors of STI history.

DISCUSSION

Elevated HIV seroprevalence rates have been widely documented in studies of men and women receiving care for a mental illness. Although sexual behaviors that confer risk for HIV also heighten risk for a host of other STIs, this study is one of only a few to document patterns and correlates of non-HIV related STIs among psychiatric patients. Consistent with other recent reports (Erbelding, Hummel, Hogan, & Zenilman, 2001; Erbelding et al., 2004; Rosenberg et al., 2001; Sitzman et al., 1995), 38% of our sample reported a lifetime STI, and 8% reported experiencing an STI within the past year. Because STIs often show few if any symptoms and our study did not involve STI testing, prevalence rates reported here likely represent an underestimate of the actual number of STIs. In a study of the general population, Laumann et al. (Laumann, Gagnon, Michael, & Michaels, 1994) found that 16.9% of the general population reported a lifetime STI. It is difficult to compare rates across studies that vary widely in their sampling and assessment methods. Nonetheless, the rates found in our study indicate that further investigation of the epidemiology of STIs among persons with mental illness is warranted.

Also consistent with broader epidemiological trends observed in population-based samples (IOM, 1997), patients reporting a lifetime STI history were more likely to be of non-White race/ethnicity, unmarried, and unemployed. Although prior research points to higher rates of sexual risk behavior among psychiatric patients with non-schizophrenia spectrum diagnoses (Carey et al., 2001; Carey et al., 2004), multivariate analyses revealed no differences in STI rates as a function of diagnosis, psychological distress, or functional impairment. Similarly, risk for alcohol and drug dependence over the last year did not emerge as a multivariate predictor of STI history, despite findings indicating higher rates of HIV risk behavior among heavy substance users (Cooper & Orcutt, 2000; McKinnon et al., 2001; Vanable et al., 2004). It may be that psychiatric symptoms and substance use patterns are more sensitive as predictors of current sexual behavior patterns rather than lifetime sexual health habits.

The experience of being diagnosed and treated for an STI may heighten awareness and serve as a "cue to action" for behavior change to reduce subsequent STI and HIV risk. On this basis, we had hypothesized that patients with a lifetime STI history would report superior HIV knowledge, more favorable attitudes towards risk reduction, and lower rates of current sexual risk behavior. These hypotheses were only partially confirmed; those with an STI diagnosis were more knowledgeable about HIV and expressed more favorable attitudes towards risk reduction, but they also reported higher rates of sexual risk behavior relative to patients without an STI history. Thus, diagnosis and treatment for STIs may increase HIV-related awareness and knowledge, but they do not necessarily lead to changes in sexual risk behavior. Theoretical frameworks such as the Information-Motivation-Behavioral-Skills model suggest that knowledge and motivation need to be supplemented with specific skills in order to effectively change risk behavior (Fisher & Fisher, 1992).

Most publicly funded STI clinics are mandated to provide risk-reduction counseling. However, with a few notable exceptions (Coury-Doniger, Levenkron, McGrath, Knox, & Urban, 2000; Kamb et al., 1998), clinic-based risk-reduction counseling is limited to didactic messages concerning methods to reduce risks for STIs and HIV, with little emphasis on skills training required to achieve lasting change. The trends observed in this sample may reflect this emphasis. As a result of receiving STI care, psychiatric patients in our sample may have experienced heightened awareness of their vulnerability to STIs (including HIV) and became more knowledgeable about HIV. However, without more intensive risk-reduction counseling, these patients maintained the same risky sexual behavior patterns that made them vulnerable to an STI in the first place.

Increasing awareness of HIV as a major health concern in psychiatric settings has led to the development of HIV risk-reduction interventions that are tailored to the needs of the mentally ill (Carey et al., 2004). Further, practice guidelines recommend that patients receiving psychiatric care undergo routine screening for HIV as part of standard care (Cournos & Bakalar, 1996). Although continued HIV risk reduction efforts are clearly warranted, our findings highlight the need for an expanded focus on diagnostic screening and risk reduction programs that target both HIV and other more commonly occurring STIs. Fortunately, several promising intensive HIV risk reduction interventions developed for psychiatric patients could be adapted for use as interventions to reduce risks for both HIV and STI risks (Carey et al., 2004; Otto-Salaj, Kelly, Stevenson, Hoffman, & Kalichman, 2001). Promoting awareness of the high prevalence rates of STIs among people with mental illness could strengthen HIV prevention efforts by highlighting patients' perceived susceptibility to a wide range of health problems that can result from risky sexual behavior.

Our study involved cross-sectional analyses that examined the association of current knowledge, attitudes and behaviors to lifetime STI diagnoses. Although intriguing, inferences concerning a temporal association between past STI treatment and subsequent changes in behavior require confirmation with prospective studies. Other study limitations include the absence of biologically confirmed STI diagnoses and the fact that our sample was limited to psychiatric patients who reported sexual activity within the past year. A broader recruitment strategy that includes less sexually active patients would likely yield lower overall STI rates.

In conclusion, the current study is one of the first to report data on attitudinal, behavioral, and psychiatric factors associated with STIs among persons with mental illness. Our findings suggest elevated lifetime STI rates among psychiatric patients and support the need for sexual health services in psychiatric settings that include skills-training to reduce high-risk sexual behavior, along with the provision of information about STIs and how they are contracted. Ample evidence suggests that sexual health services offered within psychiatric settings can be effective in reducing risk behavior, with anticipated positive benefits to patients and the communities where they live and receive care.

REFERENCES

Carey, M. P., Carey, K. B., Maisto, S. A., Gordon, C. M., Schroder, K. E., & Vanable, P. A. (2004). Reducing HIV-risk behavior among adults receiving outpatient psychiatric treatment: Results from a randomized controlled trial. *Journal of Consulting and Clinical Psychology, 72*, 252-268.

Carey, M. P., Carey, K. B., Maisto, S. A., Gordon, C. M., & Vanable, P. A. (2001). Prevalence and correlates of sexual activity and HIV-related risk behavior among psychiatric outpatients. *Journal of Consulting and Clinical Psychology, 69*, 846-850.

Carey, M. P., Carey, K. B., Maisto, S. A., Gordon, C. M., & Weinhardt, L. S. (2001). Assessing sexual risk behaviour with the timeline followback (tlfb) approach: Continued development and psychometric evaluation with psychiatric outpatients. *International Journal of STD and AIDS, 12*, 365-375.

Carey, M. P., Carey, K. B., Maisto, S. A., Schroder, K. E., Vanable, P. A., & Gordon, C. M. (2004). HIV risk behavior among psychiatric outpatients: Association with psychiatric disorder, substance use disorder, and gender. *Journal of Nervous and Mental Diseases, 192*, 289-296.

Carey, M. P., Carey, K. B., Weinhardt, L. S., & Gordon, C. M. (1997). Behavioral risk for HIV infection among adults with a severe and persistent mental illness: Patterns and psychological antecedents. *Community Mental Health Journal, 33*, 133-142.

Carey, M. P., Morrison, D. M., & Johnson, B. T. (1997). The HIV-knowledge questionnaire: Development and evaluation of a reliable, valid, and practical self-administered questionnaire. *AIDS and Behavior, 1*, 61-74.

Carey, M. P., Weinhardt, L. S., & Carey, K. B. (1995). Prevalence of infection with HIV among the seriously mentally ill: Review of research and implications for practice. *Professional Psychology: Research & Practice, 26*, 262-268.

Cates, W., Jr. (1999). Estimates of the incidence and prevalence of sexually transmitted diseases in the United States. American social health association panel. *Sexually Transmitted Diseases, 26,* S2-7.

Cocco, K. M., & Carey, K. B. (1998). Psychometric properties of the drug abuse screening test in psychiatric outpatients. *Psychological Assessment, 10,* 408-414.

Cooper, M. L., & Orcutt, H. K. (2000). Alcohol use, condom use and partner type among heterosexual adolescents and young adults. *Journal of Studies on Alcohol, 61,* 413-419.

Cournos, F., & Bakalar, N. (1996). *AIDS and people with severe mental illness: A handbook for mental health professionals.* New Haven, CT: Yale University Press.

Coury-Doniger, P., Levenkron, J. C., McGrath, P. L., Knox, K. L., & Urban, M. A. (2000). From theory to practice: Use of stage of change to develop an std/HIV behavioral intervention. Phase 2: Stage-based behavioral counseling strategies for sexual risk reduction. *Cognitive and Behavioral Practice, 7,* 395-406.

Crosby, R. A., DiClemente, R. J., Wingood, G. M., Salazar, L. F., Rose, E., Levine, D. et al. (2004). Associations between sexually transmitted disease diagnosis and subsequent sexual risk and sexually transmitted disease incidence among adolescents. *Sexually Transmitted Diseases, 31,* 205-208.

Derogatis, L. R., & Spencer, P. M. (1983). *The brief symptom inventory: Administration, scoring, and procedures manual-I.* Baltimore, MD: Clinical Psychometric Research.

Erbelding, E. J., Hummel, B., Hogan, T., & Zenilman, J. (2001). High rates of depressive symptoms in std clinic patients. *Sexually Transmitted Diseases, 28,* 281-284.

Erbelding, E. J., Hutton, H. E., Zenilman, J. M., Hunt, W. P., & Lyketsos, C. G. (2004). The prevalence of psychiatric disorders in sexually transmitted disease clinic patients and their association with sexually transmitted disease risk. *Sexually Transmitted Diseases, 31,* 8-12.

First, M. G., Spitzer, R. L., Gibbon, M., & Williams, J. B. W. (1995). *Structured clinical interview for the dsm-iv-patient version (scid-i/p, version 2.0).* New York: New York State Psychiatric Institute.

Fishbein, M. (2000). The role of theory in HIV prevention. *AIDS Care, 12,* 273-278.

Fisher, J. D., & Fisher, W. A. (1992). Changing AIDS-risk behavior. *Psychological Bulletin, 111,* 455-474.

Fortenberry, J. D., Brizendine, E. J., Katz, B. P., & Orr, D. P. (2002). Post-treatment sexual and prevention behaviours of adolescents with sexually transmitted infections. *Sex Transmitted Infections, 78,* 365-368.

Gordon, C. M., Carey, M. P., Carey, K. B., Maisto, S. A., & Weinhardt, L. S. (1999). Understanding HIV-related risk among persons with a severe and persistent mental illness: Insights from qualitative inquiry. *Journal of Nervous and Mental Diseases, 187,* 208-216.

IOM. (1997). *The hidden epidemic: Confronting sexually transmitted diseases.* Washington, D.C.: National Academy Press, 1997.

Kalichman, S. C., Kelly, J. A., Johnson, J. R., & Bulto, M. (1994). Factors associated with risk for HIV infection among chronic mentally ill adults. *American Journal of Psychiatry, 151,* 221-227.

Kamb, M. L., Fishbein, M., Douglas, J. M., Jr., Rhodes, F., Rogers, J., Bolan, G. et al. (1998). Efficacy of risk-reduction counseling to prevent human immunodeficiency virus and sexually transmitted diseases: A randomized controlled trial. Project respect study group. *Journal of the American Medical Association, 280,* 1161-1167.

Kelly, J. A., Murphy, D. A., Sikkema, K. J., Somlai, A. M., Mulry, G. W., Fernandez, M. I. et al. (1995). Predictors of high and low levels of HIV risk behavior among adults with chronic mental illness. *Psychiatric Services, 46,* 813-818.

Laumann, E. O., Gagnon, J. H., Michael, R. T., & Michaels, S. (1994). *The social organization of sexuality: Sexual practices in the United States.* Chicago, IL: University of Chicago Press.

Maisto, S. A., Carey, M. P., Carey, K. B., Gordon, C. M., & Gleason, J. R. (2000). Use of the audit and the dast-10 to identify alcohol and drug use disorders among adults with a severe and persistent mental illness. *Psychological Assessment, 12,* 186-192.

McKinnon, K., Cournos, F., & Herman, R. (2001). A lifetime alcohol or other drug use disorder and specific psychiatric symptoms predict sexual risk for HIV infection among people with severe mental illness. *AIDS and Behavior, 5,* 233-240.

Otto-Salaj, L. L., Heckman, T. G., Stevenson, L. Y., & Kelly, J. A. (1998). Patterns, predictors and gender differences in HIV risk among severely mentally ill men and women. *Community Mental Health Journal, 34,* 175-190.

Otto-Salaj, L. L., Kelly, J. A., Stevenson, L. Y., Hoffman, R., & Kalichman, S. C. (2001). Outcomes of a randomized small-group HIV prevention intervention trial for people with serious mental illness. *Community Mental Health Journal, 37,* 123-144.

Rosenberg, S. D., Goodman, L. A., Osher, F. C., Swartz, M. S., Essock, S. M., Butterfield, M. I. et al. (2001). Prevalence of HIV, hepatitis b, and hepatitis c in people with severe mental illness. *American Journal of Public Health, 91,* 31-37.

Rosenstock, I. M., Strecher, V. J., & Becker, M. H. (1994). The health belief model and HIV risk behavior change. In R. J. DiClemente, J. L. Peterson et al. (Eds.), *Preventing AIDS: Theories and methods of behavioral interventions* (pp. 5-24). New York, NY, USA: Plenum Press.

Sacco, W. P., Levine, B., Reed, D. L., & Thompson, K. (1991). Attitudes about condom use as an AIDS-relevant behavior: Their factor structure and relation to condom use. *Journal of Consulting and Clinical Psychology, 3.*

Saunders, J. B., Aasland, O. G., Babor, T. F., de la Fuente, J. R., & Grant, M. (1993). Development of the alcohol use disorders identification test (audit): Who collaborative project on early detection of persons with harmful alcohol consumption–ii. *Addiction, 88,* 791-804.

Sitzman, B. T., Burch, E. A., Jr., Bartlett, L. S., & Urrutia, G. (1995). Rates of sexually transmitted diseases among patients in a psychiatric emergency service. *Psychiatric Services, 46,* 136-140.

Skinner, H. A. (1982). The drug abuse screening test. *Addictive Behaviors, 7,* 363-371.

Vanable, P. A., McKirnan, D. J., Buchbinder, S. P., Bartholow, B. N., Douglas Jr, J. M., Judson, F. N. et al. (2004). Alcohol use and high-risk sexual behavior among men who have sex with men: The effects of consumption level and partner type. *Health Psychology, 23,* 525-532.

doi:10.1300/J005v33n01_07

HIV Service Provision for People With Severe Mental Illness in Outpatient Mental Health Care Settings in New York

James Satriano

New York State Office of Mental Health
New York State Psychiatric Institute
Columbia University Department of Psychiatry

Karen McKinnon

New York State Psychiatric Institute
Columbia University Department of Psychiatry

Spencer Adoff

University of Massachusetts at Amherst

SUMMARY. People with severe mental illness evidence significantly higher rates of HIV infection than the general population in the
United States. Frequently, the only access to health care for this population is through their outpatient mental health care providers. In order to determine how these providers were dealing with the increased
risk of HIV infection among this group, a survey of all licensed and
certified outpatient mental health care centers in New York State was

Address correspondence to: James Satriano, Department of Psychiatry, Columbia
University, NYSPI-Unit 10, 1051 Riverside Drive, New York, NY 10032.

[Haworth co-indexing entry note]: "HIV Service Provision for People With Severe Mental Illness in Out-
patient Mental Health Care Settings in New York." Satriano, James, Karen McKinnon, and Spencer Adoff.
Co-published simultaneously in *Journal of Prevention & Intervention in the Community* (The Haworth Press,
Inc.) Vol. 33, No.1/2, 2007, pp. 95-108; and: *HIV: Issues with Mental Health and Illness* (ed: Michael B.
Blank, and Marlene M. Eisenberg) The Haworth Press, Inc., 2007, pp. 95-108. Single or multiple copies of
this article are available for a fee from The Haworth Document Delivery Service [1-800-HAWORTH, 9:00
a.m. - 5:00 p.m. (EST). E-mail address: docdelivery@haworthpress.com].

conducted. The data were compared to a similar previous survey conducted in 1997. doi:10.1300/J005v33n01_08 *[Article copies available for a fee from The Haworth Document Delivery Service: 1-800-HAWORTH. E-mail address: <docdelivery@haworthpress.com> Website: <http://www.HaworthPress.com> © 2007 by The Haworth Press, Inc. All rights reserved.]*

KEYWORDS. Severe mental illness, HIV, mental health services

People with severe mental illness have been known to be at increased risk of HIV infection since the late 1980's. While population estimates of HIV infection in the United States are reported to be around 0.3% (Rosenberg, Goodman, Osher et al., 2001) reported infections rates among the mentally ill range from 4% to 23% (Sullivan, Koegel, Kanouse et al., 1999). These rates are from 10 to 76 times higher than infection rates in the general population (Carey, Carey & Kalichman, 1997). The wide range of reported infection rates among the mentally ill can be explained by the sites and sub-populations that were assessed in the different studies. The lowest reported rate, 4%, was found among a group of patients who had been hospitalized on a long-term care unit of a state psychiatric facility (Meyer et al., 1993). These patients had been hospitalized for at least a year and represent those with the most chronic forms of psychiatric illness. Given the level of social and functional disability caused by chronic psychotic illness it is quite astounding that HIV infection among this group is over 10 times that of the general population.

HIV infection rates ranging from about 5% to 9% (Cournos & McKinnon, 1997) were found in studies testing consecutive admissions to general psychiatric units. These admissions screened out patients with co-occurring psychiatric and substance abuse disorders. When these dually diagnosed individuals were studied, reported infection rates ranged from about 16% to 23% (McKinnon & Cournos, 1998).

The behaviors that place the mentally ill at risk for HIV infection are the usual ones, high-risk sex and injection drug use. While a smaller proportion of people with severe mental illness are sexually active than the general population, those who are engage in behaviors that place them at increased risk for HIV infection (Kelly, 1997). Many engage in sex exchange, trading sex for drugs or even food or shelter. Also, high-risk sexual behaviors frequently are associated with the use of alcohol or other drugs further complicating the use of safer sex techniques.

Only a few published studies have examined injection drug use among people with severe mental illness. While these studies show elevated rates of injection drug use in this population, the patterns of use are not clear. Reported rates of usage range from 6% to 20% (Kalichman, Kelly, Johnson et al., 1994; McDermott, Sautter, Winstead et al., 1994; Knox, Boaz, Freidrich et al., 1994; Horwath, Cournos, McKinnon et al., 1996). It appears that injection drug use among the mentally ill is more episodic than habitual, and that may be largely dependent on situational variables (i.e., in the company of others who are injecting drugs).

In spite of greatly elevated rates of HIV infection among the mentally ill, mental health care workers remain reluctant to assess patients for a history of risk behavior and to recommend voluntary testing to those found to be at risk. In two previous studies that examined HIV service provision in outpatient mental health care settings, only about one-third of respondents stated that they routinely screened clients for HIV risk among new admissions (Satriano, Rothschild, Steiner & Oldham, 1999; McKinnon, Cournos, Herman et al., 1999). While there has been little research to quantify this reluctance, anecdotal evidence suggests that direct care workers often underestimate the occurrence and frequency of these behaviors among their patients and may feel unprepared or overwhelmed to respond when they learn about HIV risk taking behavior. Some mental health care providers have voiced concerns that merely asking about sexual and drug use behavior may exacerbate psychiatric symptoms. They believe that broaching these topics is contraindicated in this population. In addition, the knowledge that a patient is HIV infected may raise a number of clinical and ethical dilemmas for the treatment team. Do sexually active or sexually provocative HIV-infected patients represent a risk to others? Is there a duty to warn others of the infected patients' status? Should condoms be provided on inpatient services? Should HIV status be taken into account in room or ward assignment? Mental health care providers often must assume responsibility for helping patients with severe mental illness to access medical care. Many psychiatric treatment teams are reluctant to take on the coordination of the increasingly complex clinical management of HIV infection. In addition, some of the currently prescribed antiretroviral agents also have significant drug interactions with psychotropic medications, overlapping toxicities, and psychiatric side effects (Vitiello, Burnam, Bing, Beckman et al., 2003).

Given the over-representation of the mentally ill among the HIV infected and the fact that most mentally ill persons rely on Medicaid for health care, it is little surprise that individuals with co-occurring disorders represent a significant subpopulation of those receiving Medicaid HIV care. Two studies have reported that people with severe mental illness represent over 12% of those receiving Medicaid-reimbursed HIV services (Walkup, Crystal & Sambamoorthi, 1999; Blank, Mandell, Aiken & Hadley, 2002).

In 1996 the National Institute of Mental Health convened a panel of experts to discuss HIV infection among people with a severe mental illness (Carey & Cournos, 1997). The panel put forth several hypotheses in need of further investigation: that people with mental illness would be diagnosed later in the course of HIV illness; that they would be more physically ill when diagnosed; and that they would require more costly care. If people with mental illness are identified as representing a significant minority of those receiving publicly financed HIV care, and they cost more to care for, and the front line providers, that is mental health care practitioners, are not doing what is necessary to identify those who are infected, then a number of negative health and public health consequences can be expected to follow. This study sought to: (1) describe HIV-related services being delivered in out-patient mental health care settings in New York State, including prevention, identification of HIV cases and arrangements for medical care and management; (2) compare current practices with those in place at the time that the NIH expert panel released its recommendations.

METHODS

A questionnaire assessing HIV/AIDS services was sent to the directors of all licensed and certified outpatient mental health care programs in New York State in August 2003. The 18 item questionnaire concentrated on program demographics (program size, program locale, percentage of clients with HIV and/or substance abuse disorders, client services reimbursement streams), HIV services offered (HIV risk assessment, on-site HIV testing, referrals off-site for HIV services, condom distribution), training issues (has staff received training and does staff need training in HIV service provision) and coordination of psychiatric and HIV care. The surveys were coded to assist in identifying non-responding programs. The initial mailing of 957 surveys resulted in the completion and return of less than a third of those sent. After a period of 6 months, non-responding programs were re-contacted and again asked to complete and return the survey. Of the 957 surveys sent, 392 were returned for a response rate of 40.9%. This response rate, therefore, underestimates the total response rate as some programs had closed and some large programs with multiple sites and multiple licenses responded with one survey. Which programs responded and which ones were represented by multiple sites? Did response rate vary based on program sponsor?

RESULTS

Table 1 shows characteristics of the 392 programs reporting their HIV/IADS services and training need in 2004. The majority of responding programs were urban (59.6%), although sizable proportions of suburban (22.0%) and rural (18.4%) programs responded. The majority of programs (58.2%) served over 200 clients annually with only 28.1% of programs reporting serving fewer than 100 clients per year. The vast majority of programs reported treating patients with substance use disorders with only 4.4% stating that they did not treat people with co-occurring substance abuse and mental illness. Over three quarters of respondents (76.7%) said that they treated known HIV-infected patients in their settings. Almost a quarter (23.3%), therefore, either did not have, or did not know about HIV-infected patients at their clinics. Over half (50.8%) stated that they treated between 1 and 10 HIV-infected patients annually, and 17.8% said they treated between 11 and 50 of these patients each year.

In terms of how the responding programs are reimbursed for the services that they provide, almost three quarters (72.0%) stated that the majority of their clientele were on Medicaid/Medicare. Only 2.4% of respondents stated that they did not have any Medicaid/Medicare patients. As can be expected from the above result, the majority of programs (55.8%) reported that they had only between 1% and 25% of self-pay clients. In terms of managed care, only a small percentage of respondents (8.7%) reported that over half of their clientele was covered by a managed care plan.

While more than half of the respondents (55.2%) stated that they provided HIV educational material to their clients, far fewer provided concrete services designed to identify and treat or prevent HIV infection among clients: 46.0% conducted risk reduction interventions; 21.6% offered HIV test counseling; and less than one fifth (17.0%) of respondents offered support groups for HIV-positive clients. Despite being a requirement of the New York State Office of Mental Health since the early 1990's, less than half of responding programs (44.1%) reported that they conducted routine HIV risk assessment at intake. When asked what they would do with a client who revealed an HIV risk history, only 16.2% of programs reported offering HIV testing on-site. The vast majority of pro-

TABLE 1. Characteristics of 392 outpatient mental health care agencies and their HIV/mental health services and training needs, 2004 and comparison data from a similar survey in 1997.

VARIABLE	1997 N^1	%	2004 N^1	%	X^2, (df), p
Location					
Urban	284	60.9	227	59.6	9.12, (2)
Suburban	128	27.5	84	22.0	p < 0.025
Rural	54	11.6	70	18.4	
Number of clients served per year					
1-50	35	7.6	46	11.9	
51-100	50	10.8	63	16.2	15.2, (4)
101-200	96	20.7	53	13.7	p < 0.01
201-500	120	25.9	99	25.5	
> 500	162	35.0	127	32.7	
Percentage of clients with identified alcohol or other drug use disorders					
0	8	1.7	17	4.4	
1-25	197	42.1	159	41.2	
26-50	128	27.4	110	28.5	NS^2
51-75	77	16.5	62	16.1	
76-100	58	12.4	38	9.8	
Number of known HIV/AIDS cases served per year					
0	70	15.2	89	23.3	
1-10	243	52.7	194	50.8	13.5, (4)
11-50	92	20.0	68	17.8	p < 0.01
51-100	21	4.6	17	4.5	
> 100	35	7.6	14	3.7	
Agency refers offsite for:					
HIV educational material			237	64.4	
HIV risk reduction interventions			218	59.2	
HIV risk assessment			203	55.8	NC^3
HIV test counseling			275	74.1	
HIV-positive support groups			280	76.1	
Agency provides:					
HIV educational material	320	68.7	208	55.2	
HIV risk reduction interventions	245	53.6	173	46.0	NS
HIV test counseling	125	27.2	80	21.6	
HIV-positive support groups	88	19.2	63	17.0	
HIV risk assessment is part of routine intake procedure	142	30.4	167	44.1	17.08, (1) p < 0.001

TABLE 1 (continued)

VARIABLE	1997 N[1]	%	2004 N[1]	%	x^2, (df), p
If client reveals HIV risk on intake, how HIV testing is conducted:					
On-site	57	12.3	58	16.2	9.66, (3)
Refer to external test site	189	40.9	131	36.5	p < 0.025
Refer to hospital or medical clinic	128	27.7	122	34.0	
No procedure in place	88	19.0	48	13.4	
Main way condoms distributed					
Anonymously	57	12.3	41	10.8	11.09, (3)
From a clinician	133	28.7	76	20.0	p < 0.025
Vending machine	1	0.2	0	0	
Not distributed	273	58.8	263	69.2	
Primary barrier to condom distribution					
Lack of funds to purchase them	110	31.8	80	27.4	
Policy due to religious affiliation	35	10.1	27	9.2	NS
Other policy	82	23.7	76	26.0	
No need	119	34.4	109	37.3	
Staff trained in:					
HIV risk interviewing	·	153	40.9		
Neuropsychiatric aspects of HIV/AIDS		113	30.5		
HIV test counseling	249	53.8	86	23.1	NC
Legal, ethical & policy issues		220	58.7		
Running HIV risk reduction interventions		99	26.8		
Staff needs training in:					
HIV risk interviewing	257	57.2	218	59.7	
Neuropsychiatric aspects of HIV/AIDS	334	73.7	247	67.7	
HIV test counseling	232	52.0	155	43.4	NS
Legal, ethical & policy issues	332	72.5	219	59.7	
Running HIV risk reduction interventions	270	61.1	194	53.7	
HIV-related services for clients are					
Essential	185	39.8	122	32.1	
Very important	141	30.3	117	30.8	21.48, (4)
Somewhat important	121	26.1	96	25.3	p < 0.001
Not very important	15	3.2	35	9.2	
Unimportant	3	0.6	10	2.6	
Percentage of all (not just HIV-related) client services reimbursed by MEDICAID/MEDICARE					
0			9	2.4	
1-25%			25	6.6	
25-50%		71	18.9	NC	
50-75%		122	32.4		
75-100%			149	39.6	

TABLE 1 (continued)

VARIABLE	1997 N[1]	%	2004 N[1]	%	X^2, (df), p
Private insurance/Self-pay					
0			56	14.4	
1-25%			217	55.8	
25-50%			67	17.2	NC
50-75%			7	1.8	
75-100%			42	10.8	
Managed Care					
0			77	22.3	
1-25%			150	43.4	
25-50%			89	25.7	NC
50-75%			26	7.5	
75-100%			4	1.2	
Percentage of HIV-positive clients started on anti-retroviral medications and able to adhere to regimen					
0			48	14.2	
1-25%			81	24.0	
25-50%			24	7.1	NC
50-75%			47	13.9	
75-100%			137	40.7	
Agency's HIV-positive clients have adequate access to HIV medical services					
Usually			259	85.8	
Sometimes			40	13.2	NC
Not at all			3	1.0	
Agency's integration of HIV medical services with psychiatric services to HIV-positive clients					
0 (no integration)			50	14.3	
1			72	20.6	
2			108	30.9	NC
3			73	20.9	
4 (full integration)			46	13.2	

[1] Numbers vary due to missing information
[2] Non-significant difference
[3] No comparison data

grams (70.5%) refer off-site for HIV testing, and, dismayingly, 13.4% of programs stated that they have no procedure in place to refer for HIV testing.

Despite the fact that condoms provide the best means of protection against sexually transmitted diseases including HIV, and that people with mental illness have been demonstrated to engage in high risk sexual behavior, a full 69.2% of programs reported that they do not distribute condoms to their clients. In only 10.8% of programs were condoms available to clients on an anonymous basis. One-fifth of programs (20.0%) stated that condoms were available to clients only by consulting a clinician. When questioned about the primary barrier to condom distribution within the program, the most common response was that there was "no need" (37.3%), followed by a lack of funds to purchase condoms (27.4%), that agency policy denied their disbursement (26.0%), or that the religious affiliation of the clinic prohibited the distribution of condoms (9.2%).

In terms of staff training in HIV service provision, a full 58.7% reported that their staff had been trained in legal, ethical and policy issues regarding AIDS and 40.9% reported receiving training in HIV risk interviewing. However, only about a third (30.5%) had received training in the neuropsychiatric aspects of HIV/AIDS, and about a quarter (26.8%) stated that they had been trained to run HIV risk reduction interventions for their clientele. Fewer than a quarter of respondents (23.1%) stated that they had received training in HIV pre- and post-test counseling (43.4%).

When asked about staff training needs, the most mentioned need was training in the neuropsychiatric aspects of HIV/AIDS (67.7%), closely followed by the need for training in HIV risk interviewing (59.7%) and in legal, ethical and policy issues (59.7%). Less frequently cited were needs for training in running HIV risk reduction interventions (53.7%) and in conducting pre- and post-test HIV counseling.

Regarding the rating of the importance of HIV services for mental health clinic clients, over half of respondents (62.9%) rated these services as either "essential" or "very important." About a quarter (25.3%) thought that they were "somewhat important" but over one in ten rated them as "not very important" or "unimportant" (11.8%).

In terms of access to adequate medical services for HIV-infected clients, a full 85.8% stated that their clients usually had access to such services, with 13.2% stating that these services were only sometimes available and 1.0% stating that they were unavailable. When questioned about anti-retroviral treatment adherence for known HIV positive clients, over half of respondents (54.6%) reported that a majority of their clients were able to adhere to the regimen, 45.3% of respondents reported that less than half of their clients were able to adhere to these lifesaving regimens, and almost a quarter (24.0%) stated that only 1%-25% of their clientele were able to do so. Finally, when asked to rate their agency's integration of medical and psychiatric services (on a 5 point Likert scale with 0 being no integration and 4 indicating full integration) only 13.2% of respondents reported full integration while 14.3% reported no integration.

Comparison of the data collected in a similar 1997 survey (McKinnon, Cournos, Herman et al., 1999) with that of the current data yield some significant differences. Chi square analysis was conducted on all comparable variables: clinic location; number of clients served per year; percentage of clients with alcohol and or substance abuse disorders; number of known HIV positive clients served per year; HIV services that the agency provides; does agency conduct or refer for HIV testing; are condoms distributed and if so how; barriers to condom distribution; staff training needs; and the rating of importance of HIV-related services. Table 1 shows that significant differences between 1997 and 2004 were found in: clinic location ($p < 0.025$), number of clients served per year ($p < 0.01$), number of HIV clients served per year ($p < 0.01$), whether agency refers for or provides HIV testing ($p < 0.025$), how condoms are distributed ($p < 0.025$), and rating the importance of HIV services ($p < 0.001$). Most of these changes were in the direction of fewer concrete services being provided in 2004.

DISCUSSION

Despite evidence that the clientele of mental health clinics are at increased risk for HIV infection, the response of New York's outpatient mental health clinics remains disappointing. Our group has conducted similar surveys over time. All licensed outpatient programs were surveyed in 1995; all such programs in counties with intermediate and high AIDS case rates were surveyed in 1997. Due to a computer problem, the 1995 data were not available to include in the present comparison. The 1997 study limited its sample to those New York counties that had intermediate and high reported AIDS case rates presumably surveying HIV service provision where the need existed for HIV-positive clients. The present survey sought to include even low case rate areas due to the importance of prevention and identification of new cases. As can be seen in Table 1, rural counties were more commonly represented in the current data. As a corollary of sampling all licensed clinics, not just those with intermediate and high AIDS case rates, the current sample represents more programs serving a small number of clients. Thus, the present sample may provide a more complete snapshot of HIV/AIDS service provision in mental health programs.

Several interesting findings emerge in comparing the data from 1997 with the current data. The percentage of persons with alcohol and/or other substance use disorders did not differ across the two time periods. But, the number of known HIV/AIDS cases did significantly differ, with the 1997 sample showing more known HIV-positive clients than the current sample. This could be due to the sampling differences, although the two samples did not significantly differ on the HIV-related services that they provided to their clientele. A rather disturbing record continues in the assessment of HIV risk for clients of these mental health care programs. In 1997, only 30.4% of respondents reported that HIV assessment was a routine part of their intake procedure. While this percentage increased to 44.1% in the current survey, this remains woefully inadequate to detect new infections and a breech of public trust when you consider that the licensing agency for these clinics, the New York State Office of Mental Health, requires that HIV risk assessment be part of all intake procedures.

A positive shift in HIV testing for mental health clinic clientele was found in the current data. The 2004 data indicate that significantly more clinics are either doing their own HIV testing or have the means to refer a client for such testing. Clinics reporting that they had no procedure in place for referring for or conducting HIV testing declined from 19.0% to 13.4%. This is important because of the potential for mental health clients to need specialized pre- and post-test counseling and the decreased likelihood that they would receive appropriate attention in HIV testing sites where counselors are not trained to treat people with severe mental illness.

Despite a better infrastructure for detecting new HIV infections, prevention and care services appear to have declined in mental health settings. Fewer programs report that condoms are available anonymously to their clientele, and more programs now report that condoms are not distributed at all in their programs. Despite evidence that condoms represent the best protection against the sexual transmission of HIV, a full 69.2% of mental health programs surveyed stated that they did not distribute condoms. Due to their impoverished economic circumstances, psychiatric patients are unlikely to be able to afford condoms and if mental health programs do not provide them, they are unlikely to be used. Evidence of why this may be so can be gleaned from how programs rate the importance of HIV services for mental health clients. In the 1997 survey, 70.1% of respondents rated HIV related services for their clients as either "essential" or "very important." Those ranking these services as "essential" or "very important" in the current survey declined to 62.9%. More telling perhaps was that in 1997 only 3.8% of respondents rated HIV services as "not very important" or "unimportant" while this number increased to 11.8% in the current survey. Again this could be an artifact of sampling, though the similar large proportion of urban respondents in the two samples would suggest that the perception of need would not have shifted as significantly as it has.

CONCLUSIONS

Several reasons may explain the apparent lack of interest in providing HIV-related services for people receiving outpatient psychiatric care. First, HIV does not command the kind of attention that it did in the 1980's and 1990's. The nation has become more complacent about the epidemic as the number of new cases has declined and the effectiveness of new treatments has led to the perception of the disease as a chronic illness rather than a death sentence. Yet, for many groups, these assumptions are unfounded. Those who occupy the lower rungs of our socio-economic strata not only are over-represented in HIV infections but are also less likely to be diagnosed early in the course of infection. As a result of later diagnosis, these individuals are more likely to be quite immunocompromised at the time of diagnosis and have a much poorer prognosis.

Why does this occur to the mentally ill? Why are our mental health care programs not doing routine assessment and referral for testing for those at risk? The answers to these questions are multi-determined. First, there may be a disincentive to knowing the HIV status of patients with mental illness. Many clinicians are concerned and confused about their legal obligations regarding a known HIV infected client who is sexually active. In addition, many clinicians are not familiar with the confidentiality protections and reporting requirements set out in state laws.

Second, the knowledge of HIV infection may raise difficult medical management issues that mental health clinicians do not feel competent to address. The combined poly-pharmacy of mental illness and HIV treatment can present daunting pharmacological issues that require expert consultation. Third, there is often little or no funding to offer enhanced services to a population that may require the coordination of medical, mental health and substance abuse services as well as housing assistance and intensive case management. In fact, individuals who require this level of coordinated care often are referred from site to site because no place exists to meet their complicated needs. This population requires a level of service coordination that does exist in certain enlightened places but remains the great exception rather than the rule.

REFERENCES

Blank, MB, Mandell, DS, Aiken, L & Hadley, TR. (2002). Co-occurrence of HIV and serious mental illness among Medicaid recipients. *Psychiatric Services, 53(7), 868-73.*

Carey, MP, Carey, KB & Kalichman, SC. (1997). Risk for HIV infection among adults with a severe mental disorder. *Clinical Psychology Review,* 17, 271-91.

Carey MP & Cournos, F. (1997). HIV and AIDS among the seriously mentally ill: Introduction to the special issue. *Clinical Psychology Review,* 17, 241-5.

Cournos, F, & McKinnon, K. (1997). HIV seroprevalence among people with severe mental illness in the United States: A critical review. *Clinical Psychology Review,* 17, 259-69.

Horwath, E, Cournos, F, McKinnon, K et al. (1996). Illicit drug injection among psychiatric patients without a primary substance abuse disorder. *Psychiatric Services,* 47, 181-85.

Kalichman, SC, Kelly, JA, Johnson, JR et al. (1994) Factors associated with risk for HIV among chronically mentally ill adults. *American Journal of Psychiatry,* 151, 221-27.

Kelly, JA. (1997). HIV risk reduction interventions for persons with severe mental illness. *Clinical Psychology Review, 17,* 293-309.

Knox, MD, Boaz, TL, Friedrich, MA et al. (1994). HIV risk factors for persons with serious mental illness. *Community Mental Health Journal,* 30, 551-63.

McDermott, BE, Sautter, JJ, Winstead, DK et al. (1994). Diagnosis, health beliefs and risks of HIV infections in psychiatric patients. *Hospital and Community Psychiatry,* 45, 580-5

McKinnon, K & Cournos, F. (1998). HIV infection linked to substance use among hospitalized patients with severe mental illness. *Psychiatric Services,* 49, 1269.

McKinnon, K, Cournos, F, Herman, R, Satraino, J, Silver, B, & Puello, I. (1999). AIDS-related services and training in outpatient mental health care agencies in New York. *Psychiatric Services,* 50(9), 1225-8.

Meyer, I, McKinnon, K, Cournos, F. et al. (1997). HIV seroprevalence among long-stay patients in a psychiatric hospital. *Hospital and Community Psychiatry,* 44, 282-4.

Rosenberg, SD, Goodman, LA, Osher, FC, Swarz, MS, Essock, SM, Butterfield, MI, Constantine, NT, Wolford, GL, & Slayers, MP. (2001). Prevalence of HIV, and hepatitis C in people with severe mental illness. *American Journal of Public Health,* 91(1), 31-7.

Satriano, J, Rothschild, R, Steiner, J, & Oldham, J. (1999). HIV service provision and training needs in outpatient mental health settings. *Psychiatric Quarterly,* 70(1), 63-74.

Sullivan, G, Koegel, P, Kanouse, DE, Cournos, F, McKinnon, K, Young, AS, & Bean D. (1999). HIV and people with serious mental illness: The public sector's role in reducing HIV risk and improving care. *Psychiatric Services, 50*(5), 648-52.

Vitiello, B, Burnam, MA, Bing, EG, Beckman, R, & Shapir, MF (2003). Use of psychotropic medications among HIV infected patients in the United States. *American Journal of Psychiatry*, 160(3), 547-54.

Walkup, J, Crystal, S & Sambamoorthi, U. (1999). Schizophrenia and major affective disorders among Medicaid recipients with HIV/AIDS in New Jersey. *American Journal of Public Health*, 89, 1101-03

doi:10.1300/J005v33n01_08

Schizophrenia, AIDS and the Decision to Prescribe HAART: Results of a National Survey of HIV Clinicians

Seth Himelhoch

University of Maryland School of Medicine

Neil R. Powe
William Breakey
Kelly A. Gebo

Johns Hopkins University School of Medicine

SUMMARY. Individuals with schizophrenia are at risk of developing HIV and are known to experience barriers to optimal medical care. Our goal was to determine, among a cohort of HIV clinicians, whether or not

Address correspondence to: Seth Himelhoch, Division of Services Research, Department of Psychiatry, University of Maryland School of Medicine, 685 West Baltimore Street, MSTF Building, Suite 300, Baltimore, MD 21201-1549

Grant Support: Dr. Gebo was supported by NIDA K23-DA00523. Dr. Himelhoch was an RWJ Clinical Scholar at the time this project was completed.

This data was previously presented at the American Public Health Association Annual Meeting, San Francisco, California in November, 2003 and at the Robert Wood Johnson Clinical Scholars Program Annual Meeting, Ft. Lauderdale, Florida, November, 2003.

[Haworth co-indexing entry note]: "Schizophrenia, AIDS and the Decision to Prescribe HAART: Results of a National Survey of HIV Clinicians." Himelhoch, Seth et al. Co-published simultaneously in *Journal of Prevention & Intervention in the Community* (The Haworth Press, Inc.) Vol. 33, No.1/2, 2007, pp. 109-120; and: *HIV: Issues with Mental Health and Illness* (ed: Michael B. Blank, and Marlene M. Eisenberg) The Haworth Press, Inc., 2007, pp. 109-120. Single or multiple copies of this article are available for a fee from The Haworth Document Delivery Service [1-800-HAWORTH, 9:00 a.m. - 5:00 p.m. (EST). E-mail address: docdelivery@haworthpress.com].

the diagnosis of schizophrenia affected the clinical decision to offer highly active antiretroviral therapy (HAART) to AIDS patients.

This is a cross-sectional study of a random, national sample of HIV experts drawn from the membership of the American Academy of HIV Medicine. Participants were mailed a self-administered questionnaire with a case vignette of a new onset AIDS patient and were specifically asked whether or not they would recommend HAART treatment. Vignettes were randomly assigned to include a diagnosis of schizophrenia or not. We located 649 clinicians (93%); 347 responded (53.4%). Responders and non-responders did not differ in demographics or work characteristics. Recommendation of antiretroviral treatment did not differ between those who received a case vignette with schizophrenia versus those who did not (95.8% vs. 96.6%, $p = 0.69$). Compared to those who received a case vignette without schizophrenia, those who received vignettes with schizophrenia were more likely to avoid prescribing efavirenz, a medication with known neuropsychiatric side effects (17.7% vs. 45.5%, $p < 0.01$), more likely to agree to be helped by a specialist (34.5% vs. 12.9%, $p < 0.01$), and more likely to recommend directly observed therapy (20% vs.10%, $p = 0.01$). HIV clinicians recognize the importance of recommending HAART treatment to individuals with schizophrenia and AIDS and avoid using antiretroviral medication with known neuropsychiatric side effects. doi:10.1300/J005v33n01_09

[Article copies available for a fee from The Haworth Document Delivery Service: 1-800-HAWORTH. E-mail address: <docdelivery@haworthpress.com> Website: <http://www.HaworthPress.com> © 2007 by The Haworth Press, Inc. All rights reserved.]

KEYWORDS. Schizophrenia, HIV/AIDS, HAART

Compared to the general population, individuals with schizophrenia are reported to have both higher prevalence of HIV (Blank, Mandell, Aiken, & Hadley, 2002; Rosenberg et al., 2001; Cournos & McKinnon, 1997) as well as higher rates of HIV risk associated behavior such as injection drug use or high risk sexual behavior (Kalichman, Kelly, Johnson, & Bulto, 1994). Although highly active antiretroviral therapy (HAART) has dramatically reduced both morbidity and mortality associated with HIV (Palella, Delaney, & Moorman, 1998), HAART is not prescribed equally to all HIV infected subpopulations (Shapiro et al., 1999). Clinical concerns about adherence (Sollitto, Mehlman, Youngner, & Lederman, 2001; Fairfield, Libman, Davis, & Eisenberg, 1999; Bassetti et al., 1999), and the perceived public health risk of the spread of resistant strains of

HIV (Bassetti et al., 1999; Bogart, Catz, Kelly, & Benotsch, 2001; Fairfield et al., 1999; Maisels, Steinberg, & Tobias, 2001; Sollitto et al., 2001) may limit the prescription of these potentially life-saving antiretroviral medications to HIV patients with schizophrenia (Bangsberg & Moss, 1999). This may be true even though previous research suggests that HIV infected individuals with schizophrenia are as adherent to HIV therapy as are those without schizophrenia (Walkup, Sambamoorthi, & Crystal, 2001).

The aim of this study was to investigate, among a national sample of HIV clinicians, whether or not the co-morbid diagnosis of schizophrenia would affect a clinician's decision to recommend and prescribe highly active antiretroviral therapy (HAART) to patients with AIDS. Our secondary aim was to investigate what factors might positively (e.g., help from other clinicians) or negatively (e.g., concerns about spreading treatment resistant strains of HIV) influence a clinician's decision to offer HAART therapy to these patients.

METHOD

Design and Study Population

In a national cross-sectional study, we randomly selected clinicians identified as providing HIV care to receive a case vignette of an AIDS patient for which we elicited treatment recommendations. The HIV clinicians were drawn from the membership mailing list of the American Academy of HIV medicine (AAHIVM). The AAHIVM is an independent organization of practicing HIV clinicians in the United States representing physician and non-physician specialists and primary care providers. The membership mailing list also included demographic, training and practice setting data. Seven hundred and fifty clinicians were randomly selected using a simple random design. The first mailing of the survey was sent out in May 2002, surveys were resent in July 2002 and again in August 2002. Follow-up phone calls and faxes were completed in September 2002. Nonrespondents after the third mailing were telephoned to verify that the selected participant was still active in clinical practice at the address the survey was sent. A duplicate survey was faxed to those participants whose address was verified and telephone follow-up was done that day. The study protocol was approved by the institutional review board of Johns Hopkins University.

Questionnaire Format

HIV clinicians were surveyed using a mailed questionnaire containing a single case vignette of a hypothetical HAART naïve, patient seeking outpatient treatment for a new diagnosis of AIDS. Each case vignette presented a patient with a recent history of *Pneumocystis carinii* pneumonia (PCP), a CD4 count of 180 cells/mm^3, and an HIV-1 RNA of 150,000 copies/ml. Each vignette also included the same information about adherence to PCP prophylaxis, history of injection drug use, physical exam and laboratory results. The vignettes were constructed such that according to International AIDS Society (IAS) guidelines (Yeni et al., 2002) published at the time the survey was sent, HAART was indicated. The case vignette varied the following characteristics, race (black or white), sex (male or female), and the presence or absence of a co-morbid medical diagnosis, specifically hypertension or schizophrenia. Random combinations of these characteristics produced 12 unique case vignettes. The questionnaire was pre-tested for face and content validity by a panel of three board certified infectious diseases specialists.

HIV clinicians were asked whether or not they would recommend antiretroviral treatment for the hypothetical case. If a clinician recommended treatment the clinician was asked to specifically choose which antiretroviral medications they would prescribe. Clinicians were then asked to rate how strongly they agreed with several statements. These statements included an assessment of the likelihood the patient in the vignette would adhere to treatment, the likelihood of secondary transmission of resistant strains of HIV, and the need for additional clinical services such as directly observed therapy or help from a specialist to treat this patient. The clinicians were asked to rate their degree of agreement with each statement on a 5 point scale (strongly disagree, disagree, neutral, agree, strongly agree). Information regarding clinician demographics (race, sex, ethnicity), clinical training (MD or Non-MD), clinical specialty, volume of HIV cases, year of last mentored training, as well as practice setting were also collected.

Statistical Analysis

Univariate distributions included percentages for dichotomous variables, medians for ordinal variables, and means for normally distributed continuous variables. Comparison of means was made using two-sided t-tests while comparison of percentages were made using the chi-square method. To investigate the possibility of non-response bias we used the demographic, training and practice setting data collected by the AAHIVM. Demographic, training and practice setting data that was collected by our survey but that was not included in the AAHIVM membership data was used to describe the responding clinicians only.

Separate univariate logistic regression analyses were performed to identify individual variables significantly related to our outcomes of interest including: (1) clinicians' recommendations to initiate antiretroviral therapy; (2) clinicians' utilization of HAART therapy that was consistent with established IAS guidelines (Yeni et al., 2002). Variables reaching statistical significance at the 0.05 level in univariate analyses were included in the final regression model. These models were used to estimate relative odds ratios and 95% confidence intervals and to adjust for differences in clinician characteristics. Adjusted probabilities were then computed by back-transformation on the basis of the average values of the characteristics of the outcome predictors. [14]

We conducted a sensitivity analysis for clinicians who received a vignette with hypertension compared to those clinicians who received a vignette without any medical co-morbidity. There were no statistically significant differences between the groups with respect to recommendation to treat the vignette patient with HAART or choice of HAART regiment chosen; therefore these two groups were combined to create a dichotomous variable comparing those clinicians who received a vignette with schizophrenia to those clinicians that received a vignette without schizophrenia. Responses to Likert scale statements were dichotomized to agree (which included the responses agree and strongly agree) versus neutral/disagree (which included the responses neutral, disagree and strongly disagree). All reported p values are two-sided.

RESULTS

Response Rate

Of the 700 HIV clinicians surveyed in our national random sample, 51 (6.8%) were excluded because the survey was undeliverable. Of the remaining 649 HIV clinicians, 347 (53.5%) responded. Forty-eight percent (169/347) of the responding clinicians received a vignette with schizophrenia.

Characteristics of HIV Clinicians Surveyed

The responding clinicians and non-responding clinicians did not differ significantly with respect to demographic, training and practice characteristics. Among those who responded the majority described themselves as being Caucasian, male, physicians working in an urban environment who defined their specialty training as either infectious diseases or internal medicine. They practiced primarily in a hospital based or solo practice settings with half reporting seeing over 150 HIV infected patients in their career (Table 1). The median year these clinicians finished their last mentored training experience was 1990 (range: 1959-2001).

Recommendation to Offer Antiretroviral Treatment

Overall, 96% (334/347) of the responding clinicians reported that they would recommend antiretroviral treatment. Clinicians receiving a case

TABLE 1. Demographic characteristics of survey responders

Sex	
Men	244 (70.3)
Women	103 (29.7)
Race	
Caucasian	282 (81.3)
Non-Caucasian	65 (18.7)
Profession	
MD	295 (85.5)
Non-MD	52 (14.5)
Specialty Training	
Infectious Diseases	131 (37.8)
Internal Medicine	110 (31.7)
Family Practice	48 (14.0)
Other	60 (17.3)
Practice Type	
Private Practice	121 (35.0)
Hospital Practice	111 (32.0)
Community Health	57 (16.5)
Other	57 (16.5)
Practice Setting	
Urban	254 (73.6)
Suburban	59 (17.1)
Rural	32 (9.3)
Total	347

vignette of a patient diagnosed with schizophrenia were just as likely to recommend antiretroviral treatment as compared to those clinicians receiving a case vignette without schizophrenia (95.8% vs. 96.6%, p=0.69).

Prescription of HAART

Over ninety-five percent (316/334) of the clinicians that recommended antiretroviral treatment specifically indicated which antiretroviral medications they would prescribe. Ninety-three percent (294/316) of these clinicians prescribed HAART regimens consistent with IAS guidelines. Of the clinicians that prescribed HAART regimens consistent with IAS guidelines, 51.4% (151/294) prescribed a regimen that included two nucleoside reverse transcriptase inhibitors and a non-nucleoside reverse transcriptase, another 37.1% (109/294) prescribed a treatment regimen that included two nucleoside reverse transcriptase inhibitors and a protease inhibitor and 11.5% (34/294) prescribed a regimen that included three nucleoside reverse transcriptase inhibitors.

Among those that prescribed a non-nucleoside reverse transcriptase inhibitor, 68.9% (104/151) prescribed efavirenz, 29.4% (44/151) prescribed nevirapine, and 2.00% (3/151) prescribed delavirdine. Among those that prescribed a protease inhibitor 50.5% (55/109) prescribed ritonivir/loprinavir, and 44.0% (48/109) prescribed nelfinavir.

Univariate analysis revealed that clinicians receiving a vignette with a schizophrenic patient versus not (Figure 1), and those identified as Hispanic providers versus not were more likely to prescribe a HAART combination using a protease inhibitor as compared to a HAART combination using a non-nucleoside reverse transcriptase inhibitor. In multivariate analysis, both the vignette type and the clinician's ethnicity remained statistically significant (Table 2).

Of note, clinicians who received a case vignette with schizophrenia were significantly less likely to prescribe the non-nucleoside reverse transcriptase inhibitor, efavirenz (17.7% vs. 45.0%, p < 0.001), a medication with known neuropsychiatric side effects as compared to those who received a case vignette without schizophrenia. There were no significant differences in the prescription of the two non-nucleoside reverse transcriptase inhibitors other, nevirapine (15.9% vs. 10.6%, p = 0.13) and delavirdine (1.2% vs. 0.56%, p = 0.53) when comparing those clinicians receiving a vignette with schizophrenia to those that did not.

FIGURE 1. Comparison of dominant HAART regimen strategies stratified by vignette type.

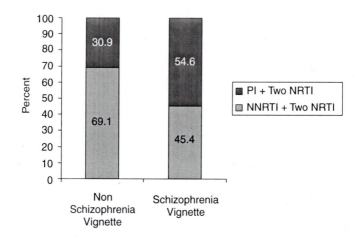

TABLE 2. Probability, crude and adjusted odds ratios of prescription of HAART comparing NRRTI and 2 NRTI combinations to PI and 2 NRTI combinations.

Characteristics	Prescription of HAART including NNRTI N (%)	Prescription of HARRT including PI N (%)	Adjusted Probability for Prescribing HAART including PI	Unadjusted Odds Ratio comparing HAART including PI to HAART including NNRTI	Adjusted Odds Ratio comparing HAART including PI to HAART including NNRTI
Vignette Type:					
Schizophrenia	55 (45.4)	66 (54.6)	53.3 %	2.75 (1.61-4.45)	2.48 (1.50-4.33)
Non-Schizophrenia	96 (69.1)	43 (30.9)	31.6 %	1.00 (referent)	1.00 (referent)
Ethnicity:					
Hispanic	7 (33.3)	14 (66.7)	63.5 %	3.09 (1.20-7.94)	2.66 (1.01-6.99)
Non-Hispanic	142 (60.7)	92 (39.3)	39.5 %	1.00 (referent)	1.00 (referent)

Adjusted for variables listed above.

Factors Associated with Prescribing HAART to Individuals with Schizophrenia

Clinicians who received a vignette with schizophrenia were significantly more likely to report that they agreed that the patient needed directly observed therapy (20% vs.10%, p = 0.01), and were significantly more likely to agree to need help from a specialist to treat the vignette patient (34.5% vs.12.9%; p < 0.001) compared to clinicians that received a vignette without schizophrenia.

Clinicians who received a vignette with schizophrenia were just as likely to agree that their patient would adhere to antiretroviral medication (53.3% vs. 48.7%, p = 0.41). They were also as likely to disagree that the vignette patient was likely to spread treatment resistant strains of HIV (96.3% vs. 95.9%, p = 0.84) compared to those who received a vignette without schizophrenia.

Of note among those clinicians that recommended directly observed therapy, clinicians who received a vignette with schizophrenia were just as likely to agree that their patient would adhere to antiretroviral medication as compared to those who received a vignette without schizophrenia (34.5% vs. 37.5%, p = 0.84).

DISCUSSION

Among a national cohort of HIV clinicians, clinicians who received a case vignette of a HAART naïve, new onset AIDS patient with schizophrenia were just as likely to recommend antiretroviral therapy and appropriately prescribe HAART as those clinicians who received a case vignette without schizophrenia. Furthermore, clinicians who received a case vignette with schizophrenia were no more likely to agree that their patient would adhere to antiretroviral medications. They were also as likely to disagree that these individuals would spread treatment resistant strains of HIV as compared to those who received a vignette without schizophrenia.

We also found that clinicians who received a case vignette with schizophrenia were significantly more likely to prescribe an IAS guideline supported HAART combination that included a protease inhibitor than those who received a case vignette without schizophrenia. These clinicians seemed to specifically avoid the non-nucleoside reverse transcriptase inhibitor, efavirenz, a medication reported to have neuropsychiatric side effects (de la Garza, Paoletti-Duarte, Garcia-Martin, & Gutierrez-Csares, 2001; Peyriere et al., 2001; Poulsen & Lublin, 2003) as compared to those who received a vignette without schizophrenia. This finding is also encouraging, as it suggests that clinicians are appropriately avoiding medication that could potentially lead to worsening psychiatric symptoms.

Clinicians who received a case vignette with schizophrenia were also more likely to agree that their patient would need directly observed therapy as well as agree that they would need help from a specialist. Again, these findings are reassuring in light of previous research that suggests that individuals with mental disorders may have better HIV related outcomes if they are receiving on-site psychiatric care (Himelhoch, Gebo, & Moore, 2002). A structured treatment approach such as directly observed therapy may be an appropriate method of delivering HAART for people with schizophrenia as other structured treatment programs (e.g., assertive case management) have proven particularly useful in this population. However, it is interesting that clinicians who received a vignette with schizophrenia were just as likely to agree that their patient would adhere to antiretroviral medication, suggesting that adherence may not be the only issue for recommending this form of treatment.

Our study does have potential limitations. Our response rate was 53.4%, however this closely matches the mean response rate for published physician surveys (Donaldson et al., 1999; Cummings, Savitz, & Konrad, 2001). Furthermore, we specifically chose a sample of HIV clinicians from a national organization that represents many physician specialties as well as non-physician clinicians which may better approximate HIV providers currently practicing HIV medicine. It is possible that there was social response bias. However, the use of clinical vignettes has been previously demonstrated to closely approximate standardized patients when assessing quality of care (Peabody, Luck, Glassman, Dresselhaus, & Lee, 2000). The design of our questionnaire, including random combinations of patient characteristics in the clinical vignettes, helped ensure that we measured the independent effects of patient and provider characteristics on physician recommendations. Finally, it is important to note that clinicians that received a schizophrenia survey were as likely to return their survey as compared to clinicians that received a non-schizophrenia survey.

Our findings are encouraging in light of previous research that suggests that individuals with schizophrenia may be less likely to receive other potentially life saving interventions (Druss, Bradford, Rosenheck, Radford, & Krumholz, 2000; Redlemeier, Tan, & Booth, 1998). Further work is needed to assure these vignette findings actually translate into clinical practice.

REFERENCES

Bangsberg, D. R. & Moss, A. (1999). When should we delay highly active antiretroviral therapy? *Journal of General Internal Medicine*, 14, 446-448.

Bassetti, S., Battegay, M., Furrer, H., Rickenbach, M., Flepp, M., Kaiser, L. et al. (1999). Why is highly active antiretroviral therapy (HAART) not prescribed or discontinued? Swiss HIV Cohort Study. *Journal of Acquired Immune Deficiency Syndrome*, 21, 114-119.

Blank, M. B., Mandell, D. S., Aiken, L., & Hadley, T. R. (2002). Co-occurrence of HIV and Serious Mental Illness Among Medicaid Recipients. *Psychiatric Services*, 53, 868-873.

Bogart, L. M., Catz, S. L., Kelly, J. A., & Benotsch, E. G. (2001). Factors influencing physicians' judgments of adherence and treatment decisions for patients with HIV disease. *Medical Decision Making*, 21, 28-36.

Cournos, F. & McKinnon, K. (1997). HIV seroprevalence among people with severe mental illness in the United States: A critical review. *Clinical Psychology Review*, 17, 259-269.

Cummings, S. M., Savitz, L. A., & Konrad, T. R. (2001). Reported response rates to mailed physician questionnaires. *Health Services Research*, 35, 1347-1355.

de la Garza, C. L., Paoletti-Duarte, S., Garcia-Martin, C., & Gutierrez-Csares, J.R. (2001). Efavirenz-induced psychosis. *AIDS*, 15, 1911-1912.

Donaldson, G. W., Moinpour, C. M., Bush, N. E., Chapko, M., Jocom, J., Siadak, M. et al. (1999). Physician participation in research surveys. A randomized study of inducements to return mailed research questionnaires. *Evaluation and the Health Professions*, 22, 427-441.

Druss, B. G., Bradford, D. W., Rosenheck, R. A., Radford, M. J., & Krumholz, H. M. (2000). Mental disorders and use of cardiovascular procedures after myocardial infarction. *JAMA: The Journal of the American Medical Association*, 283, 506-511.

Fairfield, K. M., Libman, H., Davis, R. B., & Eisenberg, D. M. (1999). Delays in protease inhibitor use in clinical practice. *Journal of General Internal Medicine*, 14, 395-401.

Himelhoch, S., Gebo, K., & Moore, R. A. (2002). Does presence of a mental disorder in AIDS patients affect the initiation of antiretroviral treatment and duration of therapy? IDSA Meeting, Chicago, Illinois.

Kalichman, S. C., Kelly, J. A., Johnson, R. J., & Bulto, M. (1994). Factors associated with risk for HIV infection among chronic mentally ill adults. *American Journal of Psychiatry*, 151, 221-227.

Maisels, L., Steinberg, J., & Tobias, C. (2001). An investigation of why eligible patients do not receive HAART. *AIDS Patient Care STDS*, 15, 185-191.

Palella, F. J., Delaney, K. M., & Moorman, A. C. (1998). Declining morbidity and mortality among patients with advanced human immunodeficiency virus infection. *The New England Journal of Medicine*, 338, 853-860.

Peabody, J. W., Luck, J., Glassman, P., Dresselhaus, T. R., & Lee, M. (2000). Comparison of vignettes, standardized patients, and chart abstraction: A prospective validation study of 3 methods for measuring quality. *JAMA: The Journal of the American Medical Association*, 283, 1715-1722.

Peyriere, H., Mauboussin, J. M., Rouanet, I., Fabre, J., Reynes, J., & Hillaire-Buy, D. (2001). Management of sudden psychiatric disorders related to efavirenz. *AIDS*, 15, 1323-1324.

Poulsen, H. D. & Lublin, H. K. F. (2003). Efavirenz-induced psychosis leading to involuntary detention. *AIDS*, 17, 451-453.

Redlemeier, D. A., Tan, S. H., & Booth, G. A. (1998). The treatment of unrelated disorders in patients with chronic medical diseases. *The New England Journal of Medicine*, 338, 1516-1520.

Rosenberg, S. D., Goodman, L. A., Osher, F. C., Swartz, M. S., Essock, S. M., Butterfield, M. I. et al. (2001). Prevalence of HIV, hepatitis B, and hepatitis C in people with severe mental illness. *Am J Public Health*, 91, 31-37.

Shapiro, M., Morton, S. C., McCaffrey, D. F., Senterfitt, J. W., Fleishman, J. A., Perlman, J. F. et al. (1999). Variations in the care of HIV-infected adults in the United States. *JAMA: The Journal of the American Medical Association*, 281, 2305-2315.

Sollitto, S., Mehlman, M., Youngner, S., & Lederman, M. M. (2001). Should physicians withhold highly active antiretroviral therapies from HIV-AIDS patients who are thought to be poorly adherent to treatment? *AIDS*, 15, 153-159.

Walkup, J., Sambamoorthi, U., & Crystal, S. (2001). Incidence and consistency of antiretroviral use among HIV-infected Medicaid beneficiaries with schizophrenia. *J.Clin.Psychiatry*, 62, 174-178.

Yeni, P. G., Hammer, S. M., Carpenter, C. C., Cooper, D. A., Fischl, M. A., Gatell, J. M. et al. (2002). Antiretroviral treatment for adult HIV infection in 2002: Updated recommendations of the International AIDS Society-USA Panel. *JAMA: The Journal of the American Medical Association*, 288, 222-235.

doi:10.1300/J005v33n01_09

Community-Level HIV Prevention for Persons with Severe Mental Illness Living in Supportive Housing Programs: A Pilot Intervention Study

Kathleen J. Sikkema
Christina S. Meade

Yale University

Jhan D. Doughty-Berry

Miami University

Susan O. Zimmerman

Yale University

Bret Kloos

University of South Carolina

David L. Snow

Yale University

Address correspondence to: Kathleen J. Sikkema, PhD, Division of Prevention and Community Research and The Consultation Center, Department of Psychiatry, Yale University, 389 Whitney Avenue, New Haven, CT 06511 (Email: kathleen.sikkema@yale.edu).

This research was supported by grants R01-MH63012, P30-MH62294 (Center for Interdisciplinary Research on AIDS; CIRA), and T32-MH2001 from the National Institute of Mental Health. We gratefully acknowledge the collaboration of the supportive housing programs and the following individuals for their assistance in the conduct of this research: Amanda Brei, Amy M. Brown, Farah Mahmud-Omer, Jacob van den Berg, and Patrick Wilson.

[Haworth co-indexing entry note]: "Community-Level HIV Prevention for Persons with Severe Mental Illness Living in Supportive Housing Programs: A Pilot Intervention Study." Sikkema, Kathleen J. et al. Co-published simultaneously in *Journal of Prevention & Intervention in the Community* (The Haworth Press, Inc.) Vol. 33, No.1/2, 2007, pp. 121-135; and: *HIV: Issues with Mental Health and Illness* (ed: Michael B. Blank, and Marlene M. Eisenberg) The Haworth Press, Inc., 2007, pp. 121-135. Single or multiple copies of this article are available for a fee from The Haworth Document Delivery Service [1-800-HAWORTH, 9:00 a.m. - 5:00 p.m. (EST). E-mail address: docdelivery@haworthpress.com].

Available online at http://jpic.haworthpress.com
doi:10.1300/J005v33n01_10

SUMMARY. Individuals with severe mental illness (SMI) are at risk for HIV/AIDS. Despite the availability of supportive community programs for those with SMI, there have been no published evaluations of community-level HIV prevention trials among this population. A pilot intervention trial was conducted to determine the feasibility of such an intervention in supportive housing programs (SHPs). A multi-component community-level trial was implemented in two SHPs with a total of 28 residents. Participants completed assessments at three time points: prior to the intervention (baseline), following skills training (post-assessment), and following the 4-month community intervention (follow-up). Results demonstrated significant improvements in psychosocial risk factors at both post- and follow-up assessments, with indications of sexual behavior change at follow-up. The community-level intervention appeared to reduce the risk of HIV among persons with SMI living in SHPs, and supports the importance of conducting larger scale intervention trials. doi:10.1300/J005v33n01_10 *[Article copies available for a fee from The Haworth Document Delivery Service: 1-800-HAWORTH. E-mail address: <docdelivery@haworthpress.com> Website: <http://www.HaworthPress.com> © 2007 by The Haworth Press, Inc. All rights reserved.]*

KEYWORDS. Severe mental illness, HIV/AIDS, risk factors, community level intervention, supportive housing

Individuals with severe mental illness (SMI) have been disproportionately affected by the HIV/AIDS epidemic. Studies have documented HIV infection rates ranging from 3 to 23% among those with SMI (Cournos & McKinnon, 1997; Rosenberg et al., 2003), compared to less than 1% in the general U.S. population (UNAIDS, 2002). The highest rates of HIV infection have been reported among individuals dually diagnosed with SMI and substance use disorders (SUDs; e.g., Silberstein, Galanter, Marmor, Lifshutz, & Krasinski, 1994). Homeless persons with SMI also have particularly high rates of HIV infection (e.g., Empfield et al., 1993; Susser, Valencia, & Conover, 1993).

An extensive body of research has documented high rates of sexual and substance use behaviors that contribute to HIV risk among adults with SMI (Carey, Carey, Weinhardt, & Gordon, 1997; Otto-Salaj, Heckman, Stevenson, & Kelly, 1998; Susser et al., 1996). Co-occurring substance abuse is common in this population, especially among individuals who are also homeless (Regier et al., 1990), with rates ranging from 20 to 75% (Cournos & McKinnon, 1997). In general, substance use is associated with sexual risk behavior (Seidman, Sterk-Elifson, & Aral, 1994) and it has been identified as a risk factor for HIV infection among adults with SMI (Rosenberg et al., 2001).

Supportive housing programs (SHPs) have become an important aspect of treatment rehabilitation for adults with SMI. Individuals with SMI often live below the poverty line and in substandard housing, and many are homeless and receive poor medical care (Carling, 1993). It is generally agreed that comprehensive integrated systems of care are needed to address the multiple and complex needs of adults with SMI who become homeless (e.g., Wilkins, 1996; Martin, 1990). SHPs provide a unique setting in which to deliver community-level HIV risk reduction interventions for adults with SMI.

Social cognitive theory (Bandura, 1986) suggests a three-component process for HIV prevention within an SHP community. The first component is HIV risk reduction skills training groups, specifically tailored to meet the needs of persons with SMI. Subsequent components involve the creation of peer norms and social-environmental reinforcement supportive of HIV risk reduction. Specifically, the second component is the systematic identification and training of peer leaders to communicate messages endorsing HIV risk reduction behavior and to develop and implement activities within the SHP that reinforce behavior change efforts. The third component is the training of SHP staff to assess HIV risk behavior, encourage risk reduction, and support behavior change efforts.

The purpose of the current study was to determine the feasibility of a community-level intervention in SHPs. We pilot tested the intervention in two settings. In both communities, a skills training group intervention was followed by a 4-month norm change intervention utilizing: (1) peer leaders to systematically create social norms encouraging of HIV risk reduction, and (2) staff training on HIV prevention strategies. It was hypothesized that the initial skills training component would lead to improvements in both social cognitive and behavioral variables related to HIV risk, and that the norm change intervention would lead to maintenance or further improvement in these variables at follow-up.

METHODS

Site Selection/Setting and Recruitment

The intervention was pilot tested at two SHPs, one transitional and one permanent, which are embedded within comprehensive systems of care in two northeastern cities. Residents living in each of these settings were formerly homeless and had a diagnosis of SMI and many had co-occurring SUDs. Both SHPs are supervised residences, located in urban communities, which provide intensive residential case management within the context of a modified therapeutic community. In both settings, residents had their own apartment within a congregate site. Both settings included community rooms and meeting areas where the research team was able to conduct intervention sessions and private rooms for assessments. Participants in each setting were enrolled in a range of services including day hospital, intensive outpatient programs, group and individual treatment, medication education and management, vocational and social rehabilitation, and health/wellness programs. In the transitional SHP (Site 1), upon completion of the program (which generally takes 12-18 months, and no more than 24 months), each individual is helped to move into independent housing in the community. In the permanent SHP (Site 2), no time limit on length-of-stay was imposed.

Participants were recruited through information presented to all residents in each of the two SHPs by a research staff member at community meetings and through individual contacts. All provided informed consent, and procedures were approved by the Institutional Review Board.

Intervention Procedures

Group skills training. A 6-session cognitive-behavioral skills training HIV risk reduction group intervention was offered to all residents in the SHPs. Sessions were offered twice a week, for a total of nine hours of intervention. Up to eight residents participated in a group intervention series, and iterations of the sessions were repeated until at least 80% of all residents in an SHP attended. Separate groups were offered for females and males, and sessions were co-led by research staff facilitators. In Site 1, half of the participants completed four or more of the six skills training intervention sessions; in Site 2, all participants completed all sessions.

The skills training intervention, which was based on approaches found to be effective among adults with SMI (e.g., Kalichman, Sikkema, Kelly & Bulto, 1995), focused on avoidance of sexual and substance use risk behaviors, consistent practice of safer sex, and integration of risk factors related to symptoms and social consequences of mental illness. The primary components included: (1) risk education; (2) personal goal-setting for risk reduction and avoidance; (3) identification of risk-related triggers and self-management skills; (4) sexual negotiation and condom use skills; and (5) relapse prevention, especially in relation to symptoms of mental illness and substance use. To tailor the intervention to the needs of individuals with SMI, program characteristics included: (1) clear presentation of information, simple language and straightforward descriptions; (2) repetition of materials to accommodate the frequent attention and cognitive processing deficits; (3) nonjudgmental staff and accepting attitudes; and, (4) realistic expectations regarding participants' ability or willingness to stay for an entire session.

Community norm change component. Upon completion of the group skills training, a 4-month community norm change intervention (adapted from Sikkema et al., 2000) was conducted. The goal of this component was to provide peer norm and social-environmental reinforcement for avoiding and reducing HIV risk behaviors through a series of peer-directed conversations and activities that were conducted at the SHP. The community norm change component consisted of: (1) systematic identification of influential residents (i.e., peer leaders); and, (2) sessions with peer leaders to develop skills to communicate HIV prevention messages to other residents. Both residents and research staff participated in the peer leader selection process. Residents were asked to anonymously provide the names of three individuals who they felt were influential members in their SHP. Research staff who facilitated the skills training groups were asked to rate each resident on a list of characteristics: dependability, listening skills, ability to work well with others, knowledge and practice of HIV prevention methods. Individuals with the highest number of votes from residents and the highest rankings from research staff members were then reviewed with SHP staff to ensure that they were in compliance with SHP rules and guidelines (i.e., medication adherence; no substance use). Three peer leaders were chosen at Site 1, and five were chosen at Site 2.

The peer leaders at each SHP were provided bi-weekly sessions facilitated by two research staff. Topics included HIV prevention information, communication skills (e.g., how to deliver HIV prevention messages to peers), and leadership skills (e.g., how to develop and conduct an HIV prevention program in their SHP). Upon completion of these sessions, research staff held weekly meetings with peer leaders to assist them in developing and implementing HIV prevention activities (within their SHP). Example activities included development of a short play on safer sex and use of small media supporting HIV prevention messages. Individuals were compensated $10 per meeting and were provided with t-shirts and buttons identifying themselves as peer leaders.

HIV prevention training among SHP staff. SHP staff were offered a 2-hour training session, addressing issues related to: (1) HIV/AIDS information, (2) sexual risk factors, (3) communication skills, and (4) HIV testing. Enhancing levels of comfort, knowledge and skill among SHP staff regarding HIV prevention was intended to create norms supportive of HIV risk reduction and to provide additional support for behavioral change efforts enacted by SHP residents. This included recognition that, despite widely held beliefs to the contrary, many individuals with SMI are sexually active and are likely to remain so even if living in shelters or community-based residences. The training included guidelines and strategies for applying the information and skills to work with clients.

Measures

Participants completed individual, face-to-face interviews at three time points: prior to the intervention (baseline), following skills training (post-assessment), and following the 4-month community intervention (follow-up). Each interview took approximately one hour to complete and assessed the following variables:

Demographic characteristics. Participants reported their age, gender, race/ethnicity, education level, employment status, monthly income, relationship status, current treatment history, and history of homelessness and incarceration.

Sexual behavior. At baseline, participants indicated their number of lifetime sexual partners, and whether they had ever exchanged sex for money, alcohol/drugs, food, or a place to stay (sex trade). At all interviews, participants reported whether they were sexually active in the past 3 months. If so, they reported the number of partners, whether or not they had engaged in sex trade, and the number of times they had had sex with someone: "after drinking too much," "I met that same day," "I met at a bar," "I met at a clinic, hospital, or mental health program," and "who was a resident of my transitional housing program." For each partner, participants reported the number of times they engaged in intercourse and the number of times a condom was used.

Substance use. Participants reported use of any of the following substances in the past 3 months: alcohol, marijuana, cocaine, crack, amphetamines, hallucinogens, inhalants, heroine, pain killers, or any other drug.

HIV knowledge. The 18-item HIV Knowledge Questionnaire (HIV-KQ-18; Carey & Schroeder, 2002) was administered; total scores ranged from 0 to 18.

Condom self-efficacy. (Basen-Engquist et al., 1999). The following three items were used to assess perceived confidence in using condoms: "How sure are you that you could: use a condom correctly; go to the store and buy a condom; and, have a condom with you when you needed it?"

Possible answers ranged from 1 ("not at all sure") to 4 ("very sure") (a = .83).

Sexual communication self-efficacy. (Basen-Engquist et al., 1999). Three items, rated from 1 to 4 (as above), were used to measure perceived confidence in communicating and negotiating condom use. Participants were asked to imagine themselves in specific situations and report their ability to communicate with their partner about using condoms (a = .70).

Condom attitudes. (Sikkema et al., 1996; Kelly et al., 1997). On a 9-item scale (e.g., "Sex is not as good with a condom"; "I would feel more responsible if I used a condom"), participants indicated agreement with each statement ranging from 1 ("strongly disagree") to 4 ("strongly agree"). Higher scores indicated more positive attitudes toward condoms (a = .82).

Safer sex norms. (Sikkema et al., 1996). A 4-item scale assessed perceptions of peer norms regarding condom use, completed for both their "closest friends" and the "housing program residents." Each item consisted of a statement (e.g., "Most of my closest friends use a condom when they have sex") with a 4-point scale to indicate agreement (a = .80).

Risk reduction behavioral intentions. (adapted from Sikkema et al., 1996). Four items assessed participants' intentions to use condoms (e.g., "I will use a condom the next time I have sex") with a 4-point scale to indicate agreement (a = .77).

Psychiatric diagnosis. Each participant signed a release of information for SHP staff to provide their psychiatric diagnosis.

RESULTS

Participants' Characteristics

Participants were 17 men and 11 women, with similar characteristics across the two sites (Table 1). Participants ranged in age (from 24-62) and were ethnically diverse. Half of the sample had a high school education ($M = 11.3 \pm 2.4$ years). One participant was married; 40% reported having a current partner. Most were not working and had a history of homelessness.

Differences across sites emerged on three characteristics. The average length of stay was longer at Site 2 ($M = 63.6 \pm 32.4$ months) compared to Site 1 ($M = 9.7 \pm 9.8$ months; t = 5.96, p < .000). Participants at Site 2 were also more likely to have a monthly income greater than $500 ($\chi^2 = 4.76$, p =

TABLE 1. Characteristics of Participants

	Site 1 (n = 14)	Site 2 (n = 14)	Combined sample (N = 28)	p
Age				
Mean (SD)	40.07 (10.98)	43.86 (10.60)	41.96 (10.76)	ns
Range	25-59	24-62	24-62	
Gender				
Male	9 (64.3%)	8 (57.1%)	17 (60.7%)	ns
Female	5 (35.7%)	6 (42.9%)	11 (39.3%)	
Race				
White	4 (28.6%)	6 (42.9%)	10 (35.7%)	ns
Black	7 (50.0%)	4 (28.6%)	11 (39.3%)	
Hispanic	2 (14.3%)	4 (28.6%)	6 (21.4%)	
Refused	1 (7.1%)	0 (0.0%)	1 (3.6%)	
Monthly income				
< $500	6 (42.9%)	1 (7.1%)	7 (25.0%)	.029
≥ $500	8 (57.1%)	13 (92.8%)	21 (75.0%)	
Currently working				
Yes (part-time)	6 (42.9%)	4 (28.6%)	10 (35.7%)	ns
No	8 (57.1%)	10 (71.4%)	18 (64.3%)	
Length of stay in SHP				
< 2 yrs	11 (78.6%)	1 (7.1%)	12 (42.9%)	
≥ 2 yrs	3 (21.4%)	13 (92.9%)	16 (66.7%)	<.000
Ever homeless				
Yes	13 (92.9%)	12 (85.7%)	25 (89.3%)	ns
No	1 (7.1%)	2 (14.3%)	3 (10.7%)	
Ever incarcerated				
Yes	10 (71.4%)	5 (35.4%)	15 (53.6%)	.058
No	4 (28.6%)	9 (64.3%)	13 (46.4%)	

.029), and participants at Site 1 were more likely to have ever been incarcerated ($\chi^2 = 3.59$, p = .058).

Psychiatric diagnoses were as follows: 54% schizophrenia, 11% schizoaffective disorder, 14% bipolar disorder, 11% major depression, 3% PTSD, and 7% other. Compared to Site 2, participants at Site 1 were more likely to be diagnosed with an affective disorder than a psychotic disorder (49.9% vs. 7.1%; $\chi^2 = 8.33$, p = < .016). Across both sites, most participants (86%) had been hospitalized at least once, and most (89%) currently received outpatient psychiatric treatment. Participants at Site 2 were more likely to be in a day hospital or intensive outpatient program

(57% vs. 21%; $\chi^2 = 4.81$, p = .028), and those at Site 1 were more likely to be receiving vocational counseling (93% vs. 43%; $\chi^2 = 8.55$, p = .003); there were no site differences in utilization of individual and group therapies. Overall, 61% of participants were dually diagnosed with an SUD. Participants at Site 1 were more likely to have an SUD (100% vs. 21.4%; $\chi^2 = 18.12$, p = < .000), and they were more likely to be receiving substance abuse treatment (79% vs. 14%, $\chi^2 = 10.78$, p < .001). All were currently taking psychotropic medications.

Historical and Baseline HIV Risk

Most participants (89%) had ever had sex; 50% were sexually active in the past year. Among those ever sexually active, the mean number of lifetime partners was 19.56 ($SD = 27.38$) and 60% had engaged in sex trade. In the past year, 43% of participants used alcohol and 39% used illicit drugs. Only one participant had injected drugs. There was no site difference in use of alcohol (50% vs. 42%; $\chi^2 = .58$, p = .45), but participants at Site 1 were more likely to have used illicit drugs (64%) compared to those at Site 2 (14%; $\chi^2 = 7.34$, p = .007). There was no association between sexual activity and alcohol use (r = .21, p = .32) or illicit drug use (r = .03, p = .90).

Changes in Psychosocial Risk Characteristics
Following Intervention

Although the study's small sample size precluded reliance on inferential statistics, comparisons were conducted to characterize the magnitude and direction of mean changes on psychosocial risk characteristics following the intervention. Table 2 presents the means of each psychosocial variable based on all participants who completed baseline (n = 28), post-assessment (n = 20), and follow-up (n = 22) interviews. Preliminary analyses found no site differences at baseline for any of the psychosocial variables (except peer norms, which are discussed separately below), so data from the combined sample was used in subsequent analyses. Paired t-tests were conducted to examine changes from baseline to post-assessment and baseline to follow-up using the means of participants who completed both interviews (n = 20 and n = 22, respectively); therefore, baseline means presented in Table 2 may differ slightly from those used in the comparisons below. A one-tailed level of significance was utilized, as

TABLE 2. Psychosocial Risk Characteristics at Baseline and Following Intervention

	Baseline (n = 28)	Post-assessment (n = 20)	Follow-up (n = 22)
HIV knowledge	12.00 (3.52)	12.62 (3.85)	13.45 (3.05)***
Self-efficacy			
Condom use	9.68 (2.88)	10.95 (1.50)***	10.83 (1.30)***
Sexual communication	10.57 (2.04)	11.38 (1.12)**	11.23 (1.15)**
Condom attitudes	15.68 (6.96)	19.81 (5.34)**	19.23 (5.88)**
Behavioral intentions	13.29 (3.40)	14.48 (1.89)*	14.39 (2.35)**
Social norms for condom use			
Peer	11.59 (3.69)	12.00 (2.88)	12.00 (3.12)
SHP resident	12.31 (3.03)	12.76 (3.03)	12.17 (2.93)
Partner norms	11.71 (5.24)	14.05 (6.61)	13.55 (5.48)

***$p \leq .01$,** $p \leq .05$,* $p \leq .10$

the direction of change for each measured variable was hypothesized a priori (Kazdin, 2003).

As indicated in Table 2, there were significant improvements in all psychosocial variables except peer norms between baseline and follow-up. *HIV knowledge* increased significantly between baseline (M = 12.00 ± 3.61) and follow-up (M = 13.45 ± 3.05) (t = 2.54, p = .010), though there was no initial increase between baseline (*M* = 12.10 ± 3.59) and post-assessment (M = 12.62 ± 3.85) (t = .87, p = .20). *Condom use self-efficacy* increased significantly between baseline (M = 9.90 ± 2.41) and post-assessment (M = 10.95 ± 1.50) (t = 2.59, p = .009), and between baseline (M = 9.57 ± 2.68) and follow-up (M = 10.38 ± 1.30) (t = 2.72, p = .006). *Sexual communication self-efficacy* also increased significantly between baseline (M = 10.90 ± 1.45) and post-assessment (M = 11.38 ± 1.12) (t = 2.35, p = .015), and between baseline (M = 10.68 ± 1.52) and follow-up (M = 11.23 ± 1.15) (t = 1.87, p = .038). *Condom attitudes* improved significantly between baseline (M = 16.43 ± 6.64) and post-assessment (M = 19.81 ± 5.34) (t = 2.45, p = .012), and between baseline (M = 16.73 ± 7.21) and follow-up (M = 19.23 ± 5.88) (t = 2.43, p = .012). *Behavioral intentions* to use condoms also approached significance between baseline (M = 13.62 ± 3.06) and post-assessment (M = 14.48 ± 1.89) (t = 1.69, p = .055), and improved significantly between baseline (M = 13.61 ± 3.16) and follow-up (14.39 ± 2.35) (t = 1.78, p = .045).

There were significant site differences in social norms for condom use. At baseline, participants at Site 2 endorsed more positive peer norms compared to those at Site 1 (M = 13.43 ± 3.39 vs. M = 9.62 ± 2.99; 2-tailed t = 3.09, p = .005), as well as more positive SHP resident norms (M = 13.92 ± 1.89 vs. M = 10.69 ± .15; 2-tailed t = 3.17, p = .004). There was no significant site difference in partner norms (2-tailed t = .17, p = .87). Across both sites, there were no significant improvements in peer, SHP residents, or partner norms following the intervention.

Changes in Sexual Behavior Following Intervention

At baseline, nine participants (32%) had sex in the past 3 months. Participants at Site 1 were more likely to have been sexually active compared to participants at Site 2 (43% vs. 21%, respectively), and they were more likely to engage in sexual risk behaviors. At Site 1, two (33%) of the six sexually active participants had multiple partners, and three (50%) engaged in at least one of the following risk behaviors: sex trade (n = 2), sex while drunk/high (n = 2), sex with someone met at a bar (n = 1), and sex with someone met that same day (n = 3). None of the participants at Site 1 used condoms consistently, and all but one reported never having used condoms in the past 3 months. At Site 2, none of the three sexually active participants had multiple partners or engaged in any of the above sexual risk behaviors. One participant reported consistent condom use, and condom use data for the other two participants was missing. At both sites, participants commonly met their partner through the mental health system (50% at Site 1 and 67% at Site 2).

Because of site differences, the sexual behavior data was analyzed separately by site. Given the small number of sexually active participants, we decided to consider individual–rather than group–level changes in sexual behavior following the intervention. An individual's behavior was considered "improved" if s/he reported a reduction in the number of sex partners and/or an increase in the frequency of condom use.

Site 1. Over the 9-month study period, eight (57%) of the participants at Site 1 were sexually active. Two of these participants were lost during the follow-up period. All of the six remaining participants demonstrated improvements in sexual risk behavior following the intervention. Two participants, both of whom had never used condoms at baseline, became abstinent during the follow-up period. Two additional participants, who had multiple partners and never or infrequently used condoms at baseline, reduced their number of partners and substantially increased their use of condoms to 84% and 100% following the intervention. The final two participants, who had been abstinent at baseline, attained a sex partner and consistently used condoms during the follow-up period.

Site 2. Over the 9-month study period, only four (29%) of the participants at Site 2 were sexually active. Three of these participants reported consistent condom use during follow-up. The fourth participant was abstinent at baseline, attained a sex partner at post-assessment with whom she had sex twice and used a condom only once, and then was abstinent again at follow-up. Because of the small number of sexually active participants at this site, it is more difficult to draw conclusions regarding changes in sexual behavior. However, it appears that the participants at this site were less likely to be sexually active, had fewer partners and intercourse episodes, and were more likely to report consistent condom use (even before the intervention).

DISCUSSION

This pilot study demonstrated the feasibility of implementing a multi-component intervention that involved HIV risk reduction skills training groups, community norm change activities, and staff training in SHPs serving individuals with SMI. Results suggest that a community-level intervention can improve psychosocial factors related to HIV risk behavior and provide indications of change in sexual risk behavior. Following both the skills training and community norm change intervention, participants reported significant increases in self-efficacy, condom-related attitudes, and behavioral intentions to reduce HIV risk behavior. Interestingly, while HIV knowledge did not improve immediately following the skills training group intervention, a significant increase was evident following the community norm change activities.

Changes in sexual risk behavior were more difficult to ascertain. While most participants reported histories of sexual risk behavior, only a portion of participants were sexually active immediately prior to and during the study period. At Site 1, 75% of the sexually active participants reported a reduction in their number of partners and/or increased condom use following the community-level intervention. At Site 2, it was not possible to determine intervention effects due to the low level of current sexual activity. Participant characteristics may explain differences in sexual behavior between sites. Residents in Site 1 were more likely to have been dually diagnosed with SMI and SUD, to have affective disorders compared to psychotic disorders, to have a history of incarceration, to have a shorter length of stay in the SHP, and to have a lower monthly income. These social and contextual issues may have influenced sexual behavior. For both SHP sites, the semi-structured living situation may have influenced the level of sexual activity reported at baseline (especially for participants who had been living in the SHP longer) and throughout the study period. Importantly, it should be noted that individuals who demonstrated greater behavioral risk for HIV at baseline (primarily Site 1 participants) did report reductions in risk behavior, and appeared to benefit from the intervention.

We emphasize the preliminary and illustrative nature of these findings. A small number of individuals participated in the intervention, the study was implemented in only two programs, the findings are based on self-report, and no comparison group was utilized. Despite these limitations, the successful conduct of this pilot intervention trial provides support for utilizing SHPs as a unique setting for implementing community-level HIV prevention interventions among persons with SMI. High levels of attendance by SHP residents suggest an interest in becoming informed about and reducing risk for HIV/AIDS. We believe that the skills training intervention was necessary to motivate and initiate risk reduction. However, the community norm changes activities that were developed and implemented by SHP resident peer leaders, with support from SHP and research staff, were likely important for the maintenance of attitudes and behavior supportive of HIV risk reduction. Although the impact on sexual behavior is unclear from this feasibility trial, it suggests that larger randomized controlled trials are needed to demonstrate efficacy and better understand the longer-term effect on HIV risk behavior. For example, as individuals with SMI transition to independent living in the community, risk behavior may occur in a social context without such community support. Thus, interventions could initially be implemented while individuals reside in SHPs and be followed over time to determine intervention effects.

Many individuals with SMI may be at risk for HIV/AIDS, and the epidemic continues to grow disproportionately among this and other vulnerable populations, including the indigent and homeless. Adults with SMI are in need of targeted HIV prevention interventions that address their multiple needs, and take into consideration the social and environmental context in which risk occurs. SHPs provide a unique setting to deliver such community-level HIV prevention interventions.

REFERENCES

Bandura, A. (1986). *Social foundations of thought and action: A social cognitive theory.* Englewood Cliffs, NJ: Prentice-Hall.

Basen-Engquist, K., Mâsse, L. C., Coyle, K., Kirby, D., Parcel, G. S., Banspach, S., & Nodora, J. (1999). Validity of scales measuring the psychosocial determinants of HIV/STD-related risk behavior in adolescents. *Health Education Research, 14,* 25-38.

Carey, M.P., Carey, K.B., Weinhardt, L.S., & Gordon, C.M. (1997). Behavioral risk for HIV infection among adults with severe mental illness: Patterns and psychological antecedents. *Community Mental Health Journal, 33,* 133-42.

Carey, M.P. & Schroder, K.E.E. (2002). Development and psychometric evaluation of the HIV knowledge questionnaire (HIV-KQ-18). *AIDS Education and Prevention, 14,* 174-184.

Carling, P.J. (1993). Housing and support for persons with mental illness: Emerging approaches to research and practice. *Hospital and Community Psychiatry, 44,* 439-449.

Cournos, F., & McKinnon, K. (1997). HIV seroprevalence among people with severe mental illness in the United States: A critical review. *Clinical Psychology Review 17,* 259-69.

Empfield, M., Cournos, F., Meyer, I., McKinnon, K., Horwath, E., Silver, M., Schrage, H., & Herman, R. (1993). HIV seroprevalence among homeless patients admitted to a psychiatric inpatient unit. *American Journal of Psychiatry, 150,* 47-52.

Kalichman, S.C., Sikkema, K.J., Kelly, J.A. & Bulto, M. (1995). Use of a brief behavioral skills intervention to prevent HIV infection among chronic mentally ill adults. *Psychiatric Services. 46,* 275-280.

Kazdin, A.E. (2003). Statistical methods and data evaluation. In A.E. Kazdin, *Research Design in Clinical Psychology* (4th ed.), pp 436-470. Boston: Allyn & Bacon.

Kelly, J.A., McAuliffe, T., Sikkema, K.J., Murphy, D.A., Somlai, A.M., Mulry, G., Miller, J.G., Stevenson, L.Y., & Fernandez, M.I. (1997). Reduction in risk behavior among adults with severe mental illness who learned to advocate for HIV prevention. *Psychiatric Services, 48,* 1283-1288.

Martin, M.A. (1990). The homeless mentally ill and community-based care: Changing a mindset. *Community Mental Health Journal. 26(5),* 435-447.

Otto-Salaj, L.L., Heckman, T.G., Stevenson, L.Y., & Kelly, J.A. (1998). Patterns, predictors, and gender differences in HIV risk among severely mentally ill men and women. *Community Mental Health Journal, 34,* 175-90.

Regier, D.A., Farmer, M.E., Rae, D.S., Locke, B.Z., Keith, S.J., Judd, L.L., & Goodwin, F.K. (1990). Co-morbidity of mental disorders with alcohol and other drug abuse: Results from the Epidemiological Catchment Area (ECA) Study. *Journal of the American Medical Association, 264,* 2511-2518.

Rosenberg, S.D., Swanson, J.W., Wolford, G.I., Swartz, M.S., Essock, S.M., Butterfield, M., & Marsh, B.J. (2003). The Five-Site Health and Risk Study of blood-borne infections among persons with severe mental illness. *Psychiatric Services, 54,* 827-35.

Rosenberg, S.D., Trumbetta, S.L., Muesser, K.T., Goodman, L.A., Osher, F.C., Vidaver, R.M., & Metzger, D.S. (2001). Determinants of risk behavior for human immunodeficiency virus/acquired immunodeficiency syndrome in people with severe mental illness. *Comprehensive Psychiatry, 42*, 263-71.

Seidman, S.N., Sterk-Elifson, C., & Aral, S.O. (1994). High-risk sexual behavior among drug-using men. *Sexually Transmitted Diseases, 21*, 173-80.

Sikkema, K.J., Heckman, T.G., Kelly, J.A., Anderson, E.S., Winett, R.A., Solomon, L.J., Wagstaff, D.A., Roffman, R.A., Perry, M.J., Cargill, V., Crumble, D.A., Fuqua, R.W., Norman, A.D., & Mercer, M.B. (1996). HIV risk behaviors among women living in low-income, inner-city housing developments. *American Journal of Public Health*, 86, 1123-1128.

Sikkema, K.J., Kelly, J.A., Winett, R.A., Solomon, L.J., Cargill, V.A., Roffman, R.A., McAuliffe, T.L., Heckman, T.G., Anderson, E.S., Wagstaff, D.A., Norman, A.D., Perry, M.J., Crumble, D.A., & Mercer, M.B. (2000). Outcomes of a randomized community-level HIV prevention intervention for women living in 18 low-income housing developments. *American Journal of Public Health, 90*, 57-63.

Silberstein, C., Galanter, M., Marmor, M., Lifshutz, H., Krasinski, K., & Franco, H. (1994). HIV-1 among inner city dually diagnosed inpatients. *American Journal of Drug and Alcohol Abuse, 20*, 101-114.

Susser, E., Valencia, E., & Conover, S. (1993). Prevalence of HIV infection among psychiatric patients in a New York City men's shelter. *American Journal of Public Health, 83(4)*, 568-570.

Susser, E., Miller, M., Valencia, E., Colson, P., Roche, B., & Conover, S. (1996). Injection drug use and risk of HIV transmission among homeless mentally ill men with mental illness. *American Journal of Psychiatry. 153*:794-798.

UNAIDS. (2002). Report on the Global HIV/AIDS Epidemic. Geneva: WHO.

Wilkins, C. (1996). Building a model managed care system for homeless adults with special needs: The health, housing, and integrated services network. *Current Issues in Public Health, 2*, 39-46.

doi:10.1300/J005v33n01_10

Rapid Assessment
of Existing HIV Prevention Programming
in a Community Mental Health Center

Phyllis L. Solomon
Julie A. Tennille
David Lipsitt
Ellen Plumb
David Metzger
Michael B. Blank

University of Pennsylvania

SUMMARY. In preparation for implementation of a comprehensive HIV prevention program in a Community Mental Health Center for persons with mental illness who are also abusing substances, a rapid assessment procedure (RAP) of existing prevention services that may have developed in the setting over time was undertaken at baseline. In addition to an ecological assessment of the availability of HIV-related information that was available on-site, in-depth interviews and focus groups were conducted with Center administrators, direct-care staff, and mental

Address correspondence to: Phyllis L. Solomon, Professor of Social Work and Professor of Social Work in Psychiatry, University of Pennsylvania, 3535 Market Street, Philadelphia, PA 19104 (E-mail: solomonp@ssw.upenn.edu).

This research was supported in part by the National Institute on Drug Abuse (RO1-DA15627) and the National Institute for Nursing Research (RO1- NR008851).

[Haworth co-indexing entry note]: "Rapid Assessment of Existing HIV Prevention Programming in a Community Mental Health Center." Solomon, Phyllis L. et al. Co-published simultaneously in *Journal of Prevention & Intervention in the Community* (The Haworth Press, Inc.) Vol. 33, No.1/2, 2007, pp. 137-151; and: *HIV: Issues with Mental Health and Illness* (ed: Michael B. Blank, and Marlene M. Eisenberg) The Haworth Press, Inc., 2007, pp. 137-151. Single or multiple copies of this article are available for a fee from The Haworth Document Delivery Service [1-800-HAWORTH, 9:00 a.m. - 5:00 p.m. (EST). E-mail address: docdelivery@haworthpress.com].

health consumers. Results indicated that responses regarding available services differed depending upon type of respondent, with administration reporting greater availability of preventive programs and educational materials than did direct-care staff or mental health consumers themselves. But overall, formalized training on HIV prevention by case managers is extremely rare. Case managers felt that other providers, such as doctors or nurses, were more appropriate to deliver an HIV prevention intervention. doi:10.1300/J005v33n01_11 *[Article copies available for a fee from The Haworth Document Delivery Service: 1-800-HAWORTH. E-mail address: <docdelivery@haworthpress.com> Website: <http://www.HaworthPress.com> © 2007 by The Haworth Press, Inc. All rights reserved.]*

KEYWORDS. Ecological assessment, mental health services, serious mental illness, substance abuse

Rates of HIV infection among adults with severe psychiatric disorders are well above the rates in the general population (Blank, Mandell, Aiken, & Hadley, 2002) and the cost of providing care for those with co-morbid HIV and serious mental illness is substantially higher than the combined costs of treating those with either a serious mental illness or HIV (Rothbard, Metreaux, & Blank, 2003). Consequently, there is increasing concern regarding the transmission of HIV and other sexually transmitted infections (STI) among persons with severe mental illness (SMI). In particular, there is even greater concern for those with co-morbid substance abuse who tend to engage in more risky behaviors for contracting these diseases, and for whom infection rates further exceed those of their SMI peers. In recent years, the published literature has documented a few effective group educational interventions specifically designed for this population (e.g., Johnson-Masotti, Weinhardt, Pinkerton, & Otto-Salaj, 2003; Kelly, 1997; Otto-Salaj, Kelly, Stevenson et al., 2001; Otto-Salaj, Stevenson, & Kelly, 1998). However, these educational prevention interventions have usually been implemented for research purposes under very well controlled conditions, as opposed to being incorporated into routine clinical care of community mental health services. Consequently, we know the effectiveness of research-led interventions, but not of provider-led interventions (Encandela, Korr, Hulton, Koeke et al., 2003). Also, virtually all of these interventions have been group-oriented rather than individually-oriented. Given that many of this population do receive some services from community mental health agencies, mostly case management, these service contacts afford individual opportunities for educating them about prevention strategies for reducing risky sexual and drug related behaviors (Eisenberg & Blank, 2004). Further, the American Psychiatric Association recommends that outpatient clinicians offer HIV risk reduction interventions as part of their regular practice (APA, 1998; Brunette, Mercer, Carlson, Rosenberg & Lewis, 2000).

To address this gap, we designed a randomized trial of an HIV prevention intervention (PATH–Preventing Aids Through Health) to be delivered individually by case managers in a community mental health center to substance abusing adults with SMI. Prior to implementing the intervention, we undertook a Rapid Assessment Process (Beebe, 2001) to document the nature of HIV prevention activities that may have already been employed by case managers when serving their SMI consumers. At the conclusion of the randomized trial, we will conduct another rapid assessment to determine what changes have occurred in the service environment as a result of the intervention in order to document the diffusion of the innovation (Rogers, 1983). This report presents the results of this baseline assessment and is a qualitative assessment of how case managers in a large urban community mental health agency address educating SMI consumers regarding prevention of HIV/AIDS and other sexually transmitted diseases as well as the extent to which they address this issue at all.

The limited research that has been conducted on whether HIV prevention services are offered to this population by the public mental health system has generally found that it is rather rare, as "providers do not actively address HIV/STI issues in persons with SMI" (Brunette et al., 2000, p. 348). Sullivan and her colleagues (1999) noted that some providers are reluctant to address HIV risks among their consumers due to perceived concerns regarding confidentiality. The public mental health system's lack of knowledge regarding their consumers' risk of HIV infections relieves this overburdened and under-funded service system of the responsibility of addressing what could be an extremely costly problem (Sullivan et al., 1999). Other barriers to addressing HIV prevention with this high risk population include outdated attitudes about the asexuality of the population, lack of knowledge and skills related to HIV issues and behavioral HIV risk reduction interventions, fears and anxiety about addressing the topic, discomfort in dealing with issues about consumer sexuality, lack of designated funding for such services, and a lower priority level than other pressing consumer safety and survival needs (Aruffo, Thompson, & McDaniel, 1996; Brunette et al., 2000; Carmen & Brady, 1990; Grassi, 1996; Knox, 1989; Sullivan et al., 1999; McKinnon, Cournos, Herman et al., 1999; Shernoff, 1988). Yet another barrier that evolved from a focus group study was that case managers were concerned that discussing sexual risk behaviors in a consumer's home or private place would be misinterpreted by the consumer (Encandela et al., 2003).

Regardless of the potential resistance to the provision of prevention services for adults with SMI by public community mental health providers, there is clearly a need to offer more systematically such education. Case management provides a logical service choice for integration of HIV prevention interventions, as it targets those with SMI, particularly those most likely to engage in risky behaviors. It is also the dominant approach to serving this population (Weinhardt, Bickman, & Carey, 1999). In addition, the types of activities required for the provision of an HIV prevention intervention are consonant with those in which case managers are already engaged. Further, due to the longstanding relationships that evolve between many case managers and SMI consumers, they are well situated to assess risk, broach sexually explicit topics that are otherwise taboo and discomforting, titrate the intervention to counter individual risk factors, assess when information has been learned, and periodically reinforce learned information.

In a recent comprehensive focus group study of mental health case management as a locus for dissemination of HIV prevention, Encandela and his colleagues (2003) found that case managers who participated in the study were very willing and interested in providing HIV-prevention interventions to their consumers. Also, they did not feel that assessing risk would overburden them, even when they had a full caseload. However, these case managers cautioned that HIV prevention services needed to be delivered within the context of the case management relationship. In other words, this service should be approached organically through the course of a conversation, rather than being forced on consumers in a systematic fashion. Furthermore, given the priorities of consumer needs, such as shelter and psychiatric stability, as well as the pressing demands on case managers' time, they felt that an HIV prevention intervention needed to be incorporated into their current practices, as opposed to being an additional service. In addition, case managers felt that this topic would be best addressed in a broad context, rather than specifically about HIV transmission. These case managers also believed that it was appropriate for them to conduct risk assessments, but with regard to education they felt others, such as therapists or health care providers would be better suited. Their role would be to link their consumers with these providers and other appropriate services.

Encandela et al. (2003) also assessed the extent and type of training for HIV prevention that the case managers received and found that case managers reported that they had received limited, if any, formal training on issues of HIV/AIDS and HIV prevention. Some claimed to have received none; others received a one-time basic information session.

METHODS

Setting

The community mental health agency where this study was undertaken is part of a hospital that serves the center of the city as well parts of the southern portion of the city. These areas are extremely diverse encompassing much of the revitalized center of the city as well as many seriously deprived neighborhoods. The catchment area served by the center is almost 100,000 people with 82% Caucasian, 18% minority, and 17% under the federal poverty level. Crime is especially high and there are a large number of institutional and social service agencies in the service area. This service area has over 50% of all homeless shelter beds in the city and a large number of residential programs for persons who are homeless as well as mentally ill consumers. The agency serves 350 consumers per day and 3,800 adults a year. Thirty-five percent of consumers served are African American. Over three-quarters of the consumers have a psychiatric diagnosis related to a serious mental illness (SMI), and fully two-thirds are dually diagnosed with substance abuse disorders.

The agency has three different case management programs. Resource Coordination (RC) is a combined broker- direct service case management program. Each of the case managers of RC serves on average 30 consumers. Intensive case management (ICM) does more direct service to consumers data collection who require more intensive supervision. ICM serves on average 17 consumers with much of the service delivered in the community where consumers live, work, and recreate. The ACCESS program serves SMI adults with multiple needs, including housing supports, as many of these consumers are or were homeless at one time. Caseload size for case managers in the ACCESS program is 8-9 persons.

Rapid Assessment Process

The methodology for this qualitative assessment employed a Rapid Assessment Process (RAP) which is defined by Beebe (2001) as "intensive, team-based qualitative inquiry using triangulation, iterative data analysis and additional data collection to quickly develop a preliminary understanding of a situation from the insider's perspective" (p. xv- emphasis in the original). The team is recommended to have a diversity of perspectives and to have both insiders as well as outsiders of the phenomenon that is being assessed. RAP differs from traditional ethnography as it is always conducted by a team of at least two individuals, in terms of both data collection and data analysis. The intensive team approach is an alternative to the prolonged fieldwork required in ethnography (Beebe, 2001).

RAP is not defined by specific research techniques, but rather by the use of triangulation and iterative analysis. Triangulation refers to "use of data from different sources, the use of several different researchers, the use of multiple perspectives to interpret a single set of data, and the use of multiple methods to study a single problem" (Beebe, 2001, p. 19). In this study we employed both in-depth interviews and focus groups, using multiple perspectives to collect and analyze data, and as a means of validation. Initially we conducted interviews with representatives of all parties connected with the case management services, administrators, case managers, the agency nurse, and mental health consumers of the case management programs. These interviews were followed by two focus groups–one with case managers and the other with the consumers themselves. The purpose of the focus groups was to obtain additional data and to validate our themes from the in-depth interviews.

The team for this study was comprised of the Co-Principal Investigator of the project, a mental health services researcher and PhD in social welfare (the first author), the Project Coordinator (a social worker and the second author), two research assistants (a bachelor's degree in psychology and the third author, and a bachelor's degree in anthropology and the fourth author), and the Principal Investigator (a community/clinical psychologist and the fifth author).

Sampling, Data Collection, and Analysis

Working with the administrator of the adult outpatient programs of the study site agency and the director of the ICM program, we selected the individuals to be asked to participate in the interviews and the focus groups. Participants were selected with the intention of roughly representing the demographics of the existing client base at the clinic, and to represent diversity regarding gender and ethnicity. For the interviews, we specified that we wanted at least one case manager from each program, and additional administrators from RC and ACCESS. Thus, we interviewed two directors, 1 male black and 1 white male. In addition, we interviewed the one agency nurse who works with consumers from all programs in the agency, not just case management. For case managers, we interviewed two black males and one white female. Besides selecting consumers to be interviewed from amongst those receiving services from each of the three programs, additionally we specified that we wanted consumers who were sexually active or desired to become sexually active as an inclusion criterion. We conducted individual in-depth interviews with two black males and one white male. The consumer focus group was comprised of eight participants (2 black females, 4 black males, and 2 white males) and the case manager focus groups was comprised of five individuals (2 black females, 1 white female, and 2 black males).

The provider interviews started with a brief introduction, followed by a general icebreaker question about the activities that they engage in during the course of the day. The interview then focused on the kind of training that existed for consumers on the topics of HIV, blood-borne infections, and substance abuse, including proper condom use and safe sex practices; whether this training should be done; and who should or should not be providing the training. Providers were then asked about the training they themselves received in these domains and whether they felt they needed the training. Finally, they were asked what kind of resources or materials they provide to consumers to reduce their risk of HIV. These included what type of training they received, whether training should be conducted, who should or should not receive training, and what kind of materials or information were provided. The consumers were asked parallel questions.

After each of the interviews, the research team assembled to discuss the content and extract themes. The outside members checked with the inside members about questions regarding what they thought they heard during the interviews. For example, one team member thought he had heard that consumers engage in prostitution and another thought she heard that consumers engaged in sex with prostitutes. Although both occur, we confirmed that in fact engaging in prostitution was the more frequent behavior.

After conducting the in-depth interviews, we continued to extract and develop themes based on reading the transcripts of the interviews. One of the team members (a research assistant) transcribed the tapes (all interviews and focus groups were taped except two interviews—one consumer refused and one time the tape recorder malfunctioned). Based on these transcribed interviews a synopsis was developed and checked for accuracy and omissions by all research team members. Using the synopsis, the research team collectively extrapolated a list of themes. The list of themes was used to inform the development of open-ended focus group questions. For the most part, the questions used in the focus groups were the same questions that were asked during the in-depth interviews, with the exception of the phraseology of providing training to consumers. Instead of asking the focus group participants about HIV "training," the participants were asked to comment on consumer-case manager discussions on the topic of HIV. These changes were made in response to concerns that arose during the in-depth interviews over the term "training." According to the in-depth interview participants, the word "training" suggested formalized educational intervention and there was concern that this interpretation may have limited the nature of responses to the in-depth interview questions. Consequently, the focus group participants responded to essentially the same questions as the in-depth interview participants, with exception of this slight wording modification. At the conclusion of the focus group, members were asked for their opinions concerning the accuracy of the list of themes developed and whether there was anything missing from the list. The entire process, from conducting the first interview to the groups and write-up of the final synopsis took one month, reflecting the utility of the RAP for these purposes.

RESULTS

As can be observed in Table 1, the four topical areas that emerged from the interviews and the focus groups were the way in which education regarding prevention of sexually transmitted infections and drug use was practiced by case managers, what these administrators and providers perceived as risk factors and non-risk factors, under what circumstances they discussed prevention topics, and the training that was received by case managers. Each of these topics will be discussed below.

The Practice of Prevention Education by Case Managers

Case managers reported that activities intended to educate consumers about prevention of sexually transmitted diseases were minimal and without formal training. It was left to the discretion of the individual case manager as to how he or she interacted with their consumers regarding these topics and each worker had a different approach. Some case managers were comfortable talking to their consumers about risk-taking behaviors, while others were not. Some case managers would discuss a particular incident of inappropriate sexual behavior or some recurring be-

TABLE 1. Summary of Themes from Interviews and Focus Groups

Current HIV Prevention Practices in Case Management
    Occurs informally if at all
    Discuss safer sex practices with consumers
    Individualized by case manager
    Individualized by consumer
    May or may not happen based on perceived risk factors
    Occurs through service linking
    Occurs during doctors visits

Perceived Risk Factors Among Consumers
    Sexually promiscuous
    Multiple partners
    Male
    IV drug abusing
    Symptoms of HIV, Other blood-borne infections, e.g., lost a lot of weight
    Identified as HIV+
    Having Hepatitis
    Sexually "inappropriate" and acting out
    Engaging in prostitution
    Having a new girlfriend or boyfriend

Perceived Protective Factors
    Sexually inactive
    Elderly
    Female

Barriers to Discussion of Risk
    Southeast Asian–sex taboo topic
    Poor relationship with consumer
    Consumer very paranoid
    Cross gender pairing of CM & consumer

Recommendations for Training of Case Managers
    Basic information as part of orientation to CM
    Periodic lectures by experts–voluntary attendance
    Requirement for standard precautions of handling bodily fluids–OSHA training

havior such as unprotected sex with the consumer. For example, as one case manager explained, "Many of our consumers engage in prostitution, and we will suggest safe sex methods. But because sex is such a touchy subject, a lot of consumers just do not discuss these topics, unless they have a complaint about a symptom. This will then provide an opportunity to engage the consumer in a discussion about preventive behaviors."

In contrast, administrators suggested that was training made available to case managers regarding HIV prevention and risk behaviors, and that prevention with consumers was indeed taking place at the agency. Administrators noted that they encourage staff to educate consumers, but

"Consumers are not strong cognitively. They just want treatment and not education." Further, one stated, "We're professionals that give advice on substance abuse. When we get into AIDS and blood-borne infections, we don't know what we're talking about and are less likely to go in there." One of the administrators whom we interviewed was concerned that case managers would not have the time to deliver an educational intervention on sexually transmitted infections. This person felt that there were many other higher priorities with which the case managers had to be concerned. They suggested that substance abuse is a topic with which case managers are more comfortable and have more training and resources available in this service domain. Case management services are designed to connect consumers with resources such as a public health center. Many felt other health professionals were better equipped to address topics relating to sexual behaviors than were they. One case manager stated, "I don't have expertise in this area, so I refer to the docs. We have a lot of resources to link our consumers to."

A case manager indicated that a lot of the consumers are positive for Hepatitis C, and many admit that they may have contracted Hepatitis C from unprotected sex. Once case managers find out that a consumer is infected, they can have a discussion on HIV risk and the need to get tested. When someone gets diagnosed with HIV, case managers do get involved, making sure the consumer follows-up with medical appointments and continues with the full course of treatment. This may also trigger other consumers to request information and to begin to protect themselves from the disease.

It was also noted that education on these issues is not a priority. "We have the chronically homeless and we have a lot of consumers that do extended periods of time inpatient. We're pretty much focused on stabilizing their mental state–that's the priority–then we try to work on everything else." Or, as another case manager said "We don't have anything established to do it. I'd have to go through my supervisor and make arrangements. If we had a program in place it would make it so much easier. When you think of all the ongoing issues, sitting down and showing a consumer how to use a condom, it's not on the first to-do list. It's not that safe sex is not important, but just trying to get them stable mentally enough to be in one place to work with them, I think that's something that's generally overlooked."

Consumers also noted that case managers rarely ask about sexual activities, about having safety products for sexual activities, and getting tested. Some consumers noted that they received training on these topics from other programs and agencies and didn't need anything more as they were already knowledgeable. If consumers ask about getting examined or tested, case managers will schedule an appointment. One consumer noted that no education was done, "Nothing outside of always be safe and use protection when having sex."

Perceived Risk Factors

Training depends on the behavior of the individual consumer. If the consumer is known to engage in risky behaviors or in promiscuous behavior then conversations regarding education about prevention will surface more than with other consumers. The factors associated with risky behaviors that were identified included being male, using drugs particularly intravenous drugs, having multiple sex partners, engaging in sexually inappropriate behavior, engaging in prostitution, or having a new girlfriend or boyfriend. In addition, symptoms of HIV or another STI are other indicators that require immediate responses from case managers. One case manager stated, "More than likely training would be for someone who's already diagnosed."

Perceived Non-Risk Factors

Consumers as well as staff felt that if consumers were not sexually active, there was no need to provide them with educational training on prevention and risk behaviors. Others thought that individuals who were elderly did not have a need for this type of training. Some felt that women were at less of a risk than men. Consumers felt that any training on these types of topics should be based on consumer choice.

Circumstances Under Which Not to Discuss These Issues

There were circumstances under which providers felt that HIV prevention was inappropriate and other circumstances where they were not comfortable about discussing these topics. Some suggested that cross-gender pairing of the worker and the consumer may render conversations about sexual issues inappropriate. One case manager provided an example of a consumer who reported that she had been raped by a black man (he did not know if this was true or not), but the case manager felt that, as a black man himself, it was not an appropriate topic to discuss with her. Other workers noted that it was also inappropriate to discuss these topics when consumers were highly paranoid or in an unstable state. In addition, some case managers expressed concern that their relationships with their consumers were not strong enough to include discussions of sexual behaviors.

Training of Case Managers

Case managers received virtually no training regarding information on sexually transmitted diseases. There was a centralized orientation for all new case managers provided by the county training program. As a part of the orientation training, new case managers were given some basic information on sexually transmitted diseases. This training program also sponsors ongoing training for the public mental health system. Although they may offer a session on this topic during a particular year, attendance at these sessions is voluntary. Also, since this particular community mental health center was part of a hospital, all staff were required to take Occupational Safety and Health Agency (OSHA) training every year. One section of this computerized training was on standard precautions, including safety and handling of bodily fluids and related apparatus. Other than these trainings, there were no other specialized educational requirements or opportunities regarding sexually transmitted diseases. One case manager volunteered at an agency that did educational training in HIV prevention and she reported training some of her consumers. She also reported being asked questions by other case managers about HIV prevention.

Ecological Assessment

As a part of the RAP, we observed the environment to see if there were any HIV prevention materials available, such as posters on walls, brochures, or other information. There were none. We also asked whether there were condoms available to give to consumers. The responses were very inconsistent. A few thought that the nurse may have condoms, while others did not know and others said none were available at the agency. The nurse indicated that there were a limited number of condoms available at one time but currently there were none.

CONCLUSIONS

The results of the RAP confirm the findings of the Encandela et al. (2003) study regarding the delivery of HIV prevention education by case managers. Essentially, formalized training on this topic by case managers is extremely rare. Those case management consumers who are perceived to be at high risk of contracting sexually transmitted infections or are already infected might receive some discussion and advice on engaging in safe sex practices. Administrators reported greater availability and use of services than did case managers or consumers. Case managers thought there were greater priorities meeting consumers' primary needs for housing and benefits, and ensuring stabilization of their psychiatric symptoms that took precedence over educating their consumers about sexually transmitted infections. What also came through in this assessment was the disconnect between the willingness of consumers and the apparent discomfort of case managers regarding discussions related to sexual health issues. The barriers to addressing HIV prevention lie primarily with the attitudes of the case managers, since the consumers displayed a great deal of openness and willingness to address issues of sexuality and risk behaviors during the focus groups.

Case managers did feel that HIV and general STI prevention education was important for their consumers and did need to occur. However, these case managers did not feel that they were the most appropriate ones to deliver the intervention. Some noted that other types of providers, such as doctors and nurses, were better suited as educators on these topics related to sexual health and other risk behaviors. Several case managers resounded that linkage was chiefly their role with consumers.

Clearly, when this type of education is left to the idiosyncratic discretion of case managers, there are many who could benefit from such preventive measures who will not receive them. The failure to use existing relationships between case managers and mental health consumers to provide education regarding sexual transmitted infections is a missed opportunity for a highly vulnerable population. It is our assertion that the case manager-consumer relationship is a natural locus of intervention for risk reduction education. Further, we believe that case managers can work on the basic needs of consumers and maintain professional and caring relationships, while delivering complete and accurate information on safer sex and risk reduction behaviors. However, care needs to be taken with design of the intervention to ensure that it fits the nature of case management service delivery. Training case managers to implement preventive interventions must address the attitudinal barriers expressed by some case managers.

REFERENCES

American Psychiatric Association. AIDS Program Office (Sept 1998). *Position Statement and Policy Guidelines on AIDS and HIV Disease.* Washington, D.C..

Arruffo, J., Thompson, R. McDaniel, J.S., Sacco, J. et al. (1996). Training programs for staff. In Cournos, F., Bakalar, N. (eds.) *AIDS and People with Severe Mental Illness: A Handbook for Mental Health Professionals.* New Haven: Yale University Press.

Beebe, J. (2001). *Rapid Assessment Process.* Walnut Creek, Altamira Press.

Blank, M.B., Mandell, D.S. Aiken, L.H., & Hadley, T.R. (2002). Co-Occurrence of HIV and serious mental illness among Medicaid recipients. *Psychiatric Services,* Vol 53(7), 868-873.

Brunette, M., Mercer, C., Carlson, C., Rosenberg, S., & Lewis, B. (2000). HIV-related services for persons with severe mental illness: Policy and practice in New Hampshire community mental health. *Journal of Behavioral Health Services & Research,* 27, 347-353.

Carmen, E., & Brady, S. (1990). AIDS risk and prevention for the chronic mentally ill. *Canadian Journal of Psychiatry,* 44, 652-657.

Eisenberg, M.M., & Blank, M.B. (2004). HIV and serious mental illness: Prevalence and treatment issues. *Harvard Health Policy Review,* Fall.

Encandela, J., Korr, W., Hulton, K., Koeske, G., Klinkenberg, W.D., Otto-Salaj, L, Silvestre, A., & Wright, W. (2003). Mental health case management as a locus for HIV prevention: Results from case-manager focus groups. *The Journal of Behavioral Health Services & Research,* 30, 418-432.

Grassi, L. (1996) Risk of HIV infection in psychiatrically ill patients. *AIDS Care,* 8, 103-116.

Johnson-Masotti, A., Weinhardt, L., Pinkerton, S., & Otto-Salaj, L. (2003). Efficacy and cost-effectiveness of the first generation of HIV prevention interventions for people with severe and persistent mental illness. *The Journal of Mental Health Policy and Economics,* 6, 23-35.

Kelly, J. (1997). HIV risk reduction interventions for persons with severe mental illness. *Clinical Psychology Review,* 17, 293-309.

Knox, M. (1989). Community health's role in the AIDS crisis. *Community Mental Health Journal,* 25, 185-196.

McKinnon, K., Cournos, F., Herman, R., Satriano, J., Silver, B., & Puello, I. (1999). AIDS-related services and training in outpatient mental health care: Agencies in New York. *Psychiatric Services,* 50, 1225-1228.

Otto-Salaj, L., Stevenson, L., & Kelly, J. (1998). Implementing cognitive behavioral AIDS/HIV risk reduction group interventions in community mental health settings that serve people with serious mental illness. *Psychiatric Rehabilitation Journal,* 21, 394-404.

Otto-Salaj, L., Kelly, J., & Stevenson, C. et al. (2001) Outcomes of a randomized small-group HIV prevention intervention trial for people with serious mental illness. *Community Mental Health Journal,* 37, 123-144.

Rogers, E.M. (1983). *Diffusion of Innovations.* New York, Free Press.

Rothbard, A. B., Metraux, S., & Blank, M.B. (2003). Cost of Care for Medicaid Recipients With Serious Mental Illness and HIV Infection or AIDS. *Psychiatric Services,* Vol.54 (9), 1240-1246.

Shernoff, M. (1988) . Integrating safer-sex counseling into social work practice. *Social Casework: The Journal of Contemporary Social Work,* 69, 334-339.

Sullivan, G., Koegel, P., Kanouse, D., Cournos, F., Mckinnon, K., Young, A., & Bean, D. (1999). HIV and people with serous mental illness: The Public sector's role in reducing HIV risk and improving care. *Psychiatric Services,* 50, 648-652.

Weinhardt, L. Brickham, N., & Carey, M. (1999). Sexual coercion among women living with a severe and persistent mental illness: Review of the literature and recommendations for mental health providers. *Aggression and Violent Behavior,* 4, 307-317.

doi:10.1300/J005v33n01_11

Index